PILATES FOR ATHLETES

SEAN VIGUE

PILATES

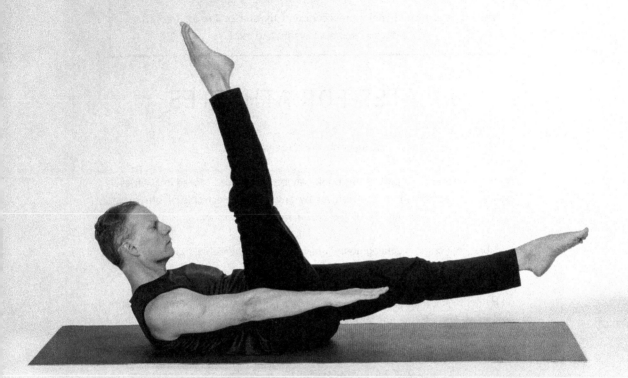

FOR ATHLETES

More than 200 Exercises and Flows to
Improve Performance in Any Sport

SEAN VIGUE

PILATES FOR ATHLETES

Text copyright © 2021 Sean Vigue

Library of Congress Cataloging-in-Publication Data is available upon request.
ISBN 978-1-57826-838-2

All Hatherleigh Press titles are available for bulk purchase, special promotions, and premiums. For information about reselling and special purchase opportunities, please call 1-800-528-2550 and ask for the Special Sales Manager.

Cover and Interior Design by Carolyn Kasper
Images courtesy of Kelly Joyce Photography

04 2022

Printed in the United States

To the memory of my beautiful dad,

Robert Donald Vigue:

I love you, always and forever.

Until we meet again.

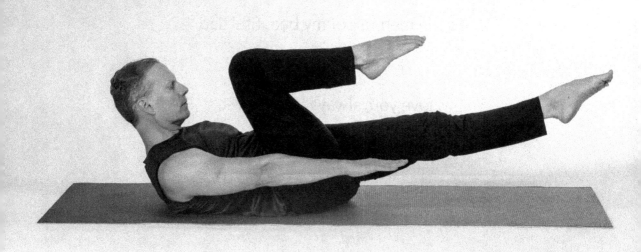

Contents

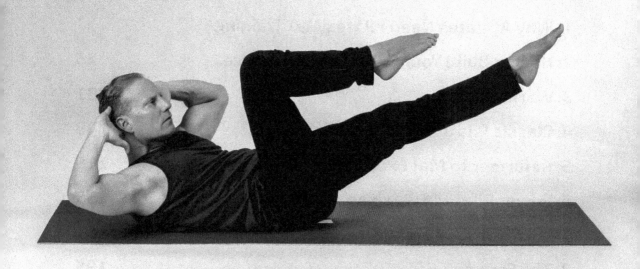

Preface

"Lower! Go *lower*, Sean!"

The choreographer was yelling at me, as I struggled to squat lower and lower into what I now call "the Russian Dance of Death" from *Fiddler on the Roof*. It was 2004, and I was in rehearsals for this classic show at the Actor's Playhouse in Coral Gables, Florida, when I found myself thrown into a horrendous dance number which involves squatting low and then popping up with great force, all while keeping your arms crossed and maintaining a pleasant look on your face. The more we practiced, the more I felt my legs and back getting exhausted.

"Lower, Sean! Go lower and jump up faster!" she yelled again.

All at once I heard and felt a *POP* in my lower back—which was not supposed to happen. It was the kind of *POP* which you know immediately is not going to disappear after a few seconds or go away on its own. Nope, that was the kind of *POP* a serious strain makes, and I knew right away I was in trouble.

For weeks, I would attend rehearsals only to lay in the aisle of the theater while everyone else sang, danced and stepped over me—including the choreographer, who seemed to be oblivious to my newfound aching and sedentary condition.

Lying on my back whenever I could, walking hunched over . . . I felt 100 years old. I felt inadequate. I felt depressed. I had just finished three months doing a production of "West Side Story" a few weeks earlier that had me lifting weights every day. I was feeling in tip top shape without a hint of back issues.

How did it come to this? Why had it come to this? And how could I fix this—*and* make sure it never happened again?

My name is Sean Vigue, and this is how I came to be introduced to Pilates . . . and how the book you're holding came to be. If you would've asked me then if I was a fit and healthy person—if I trained every day to stay fit and healthy—I would have told you emphatically, "Yes!" I was *addicted* to the gym. If I didn't make a daily pilgrimage to the gym, I would feel inadequate, out of shape, pointless, sad, you name it. When I was traveling for my professional theater jobs, one of the first things I would do upon arriving in a new location was to find and join a local gym. I loved to strength train with weights; in fact, that's all I ever did. It wasn't until I hurt my back that I realized a piece of my training was severely lacking.

My conditioning was inadequate in three crucial areas: 1) core training, 2) flexibility training, and 3) mobility training. Long story short, I was not training my body to move in a graceful, fluid way and as a result, when faced with a new way of moving—the Russian Dance of Death—my limited core strength, flexibility and mobility talents were not sufficient enough to withstand the strain, and my body reacted by seizing up and not permitting me to continue. It's very difficult for your body to lie to you . . . and mine was screaming at the top of its lungs that I needed to change my fitness ways. The days of coasting on my youth were over. It was time to take charge so this wouldn't happen again.

The style of Pilates featured in this book is referred to as Pilates mat. Pilates mat is just as the title implies: Pilates workouts using only an exercise mat. No equipment, no apparatus, no machines—only your bodyweight is needed for these exercises, workouts and flows.

When I injured my back, I had only briefly heard of this training program called Pilates (I didn't even know if I was pronouncing it correctly). The only mention I'd heard up to that point was at the Broadway Dance Center in New York where I would take jazz classes in between my theater gigs to stay limber and improve my poor dancing skills. (I was a "park and bark" kind of guy—meaning I preferred to plant my feet, stand tall and deliver my lines or songs with great strength, volume and gusto.)

So, no surprise: I attended my first Pilates mat class and was struck by three things: 1) I lacked body control, 2) my core (abs, low back, glutes, hips . . . in other words, the center of my body and the source of all power and support) was weak and imbalanced, and 3) I was in *love* with this new way of moving. I had never experienced a workout like this. The emphasis was all on things I never much thought about before: namely, good form, breath, fluid movements, constant improvement through a particular exercise, and a large dose of endurance training.

It's rather difficult for me to put into words how I felt during and after that first class. The feeling was overwhelming. This is because *watching* Pilates and *doing* Pilates are a universe apart. Watching someone perform the Pilates 100 exercise has nothing to do with getting on the mat, extending your legs, pumping your arms to a 5-count rhythm, all while stabilizing your core, lifting your legs and tightening your abs on the exhales. When all these actions are mixed into one purpose-filled exercise, the amount of exertion, release, challenge and enjoyment is . . . well, indescribable.

I began to train my fellow actors in Pilates and core strengthening to keep us healthy through endless rehearsals and 8–10 shows per week. Singing, dancing and moving on stage requires a lot of control and spatial awareness, and Pilates was perfect for helping us hone these skills. We found we had so much more energy for performances now, because we were no longer suffering from the energy depletion of poor posture, shallow breathing and a compressed body from lack of flexibility.

Eventually, I was teaching and building my *own* Pilates classes for whomever wanted to attend—power lifters, desk jockeys, triathletes, dancers, golfers, former athletes, couch potatoes, weightlifters, stay-at-home moms, coaches . . . the list goes on and on. If you came to class, I would make sure you worked to your level. Pilates is extremely versatile that way; it meets you exactly where your mind and body are waiting. It guides you. It pushes you with a firm gentleness. It wins you over on those days when you absolutely *don't* want to train. It is a conditioning partner for life. It is *yours*.

Now to this book. It says it right there on the cover: we're talking directly to the athletes for this one. Let me state up front that this book—and the Pilates method—is **essential for athletes of any sport and level of fitness**. And in fact, Pilates machines and apparatus have started to make huge inroads in the training of athletes . . . but Pilates mat has yet to properly break through. In my experience teaching Pilates to athletes, I have witnessed runners rehab and heal imbalance injuries; football players build a stronger, more balanced core to increase their speed; hockey players ratchet up their endurance; golfers tack on added flexibility, strength and control to their backswing; and skiers improve the power of their directional changes. There is no sport on Earth which I have not seen firsthand (and through my online videos) be massively benefitted by a regular Pilates mat practice.

So. Do you define yourself as an athlete? Are you someone who wants to constantly improve at their craft? Are you able to participate in your favorite sports and activities while giving 100 percent? I define anyone who enjoys a sport as an athlete. Perhaps you play golf every other weekend or are a forward in the NBA? You're an athlete. You have a passion for your sport, one that includes constantly improving your mental and physical conditioning to realize your potential? You're an athlete. You want to be your very best whenever you step onto the court, rink, field, track, course, slope, mat, base, road, etc.? You're an athlete.

And now you hold in your hands your personal on-the-go Pilates training manual—one which contains all the original exercises from Joseph Pilates, along with modifications and add-ons to fit your personal fitness level. If that's not enough (and it's plenty), this book also is packed with warm-up exercises, Pilates reformer exercises (a machine which consists of a sliding carriage with springs, bars and straps) translated for the mat, a Power Pilates section to up your training with challenging variations, and even some Power Yoga (another movement passion of mine). All this, as well as cool down stretches for deep release and a *massive* amount of Pilates workouts to get you moving and reaping the immediate benefits of Pilates.

My goal is for every athlete of every sport, age and fitness level to ignite their training with Pilates. Regular Pilates practice builds and improves flexibility, core and overall muscular strength, focus, balance, endurance and control. Not an hour goes by without me mentioning Pilates to someone—*and* why they need it right now. Someone always needs Pilates. *You* need Pilates, or else you wouldn't have read this far!

I know you. You like to move, build, create and improve. You're competitive. You want to dominate. You want *more*. You want to be *better*. But talk is cheap so let's ignite your athletic training together. Are you ready? Take a deep breath and turn the page . . . or else jump ahead to Chapter 3 and put your Pilates studies into action right now. Either way, let's get started!

How to Use
This Book

My main objective with *Pilates for Athletes* is to get you on the mat—moving, breathing and flowing—*right now*. This book is designed for athletes of all fitness levels and ages who dewsire the addition of Pilates mat to their training. This is because Pilates meets you where you are. *You* are always in control, not the exercises. These are *your* exercises, flows and training logs. Take control of them when your body is ready.

You have three options for how to proceed with your Pilates training using this book. All three will work wonders for total body conditioning if you follow them with discipline, practice and consistency. I also recommend that you read through the introduction and the first two chapters to gain a better understanding of who I am, what Pilates mat training is all about, and why is it so important for any athlete to incorporate the basic principles of Pilates training into their regimen.

Method 1: Learn all the exercises first.

Take on about 10 exercises each day to prevent overload and frustration and concentrate on mastering each one before proceeding to the next. Begin in Chapter 3 and work your way through the warm-ups into the classic mat exercises. Use the descriptions and photos to practice the exercises and advance to the Add-ons when your body is ready for more. If you feel yourself struggling with certain exercises, switch to the modification and practice. Control of each move is paramount before moving on.

Continuing to Chapter 4, you'll encounter reformer exercises translated to the mat. Work your way through them, savoring the challenge and uniqueness of each exercise, before progressing to the Power Pilates exercises. These build on everything you've learned up to this point and pushes you into new areas of balance, cardio conditioning and stamina.

Finally, turn to the cool down stretches and work on marrying your breath and movement for effective flexibility training. Now, you can move onto whichever flows in Chapters 5 and 6 you wish.

METHOD 2: Jump to your sport.

Say you're a hockey player (or any sport contained in this book) and want to know the best Pilates mat workout for you to do, right now, to improve your skating speed, slap shot force and agility on the ice. Go ahead! Flip to the hockey section in the training logs (Chapter 6) and practice the recommended routine. Each exercise has its page number listed so you can practice each individual exercise before putting them all together. Practice the flow until your body begins to get bored and then you know it's time to move on. From here, you can practice individual exercises (Chapters 3 and 4) or move into the appropriate flows (Chapter 5) or other training logs (Chapter 6). This book is a complete, on-the-go training manual, so feel free to explore and discover something new and challenging every day.

METHOD 3: Pick a flow according to your fitness and conditioning level.

If you're looking for a specific flow which corresponds to your current strength and flexibility level, flip to Chapter 5 and choose a sequence. There are 20 complete Pilates workouts, categorized by athletic level, time of day, specific body areas, endurance and the official *Pilates for Athletes* flow (the pinnacle class of this book). Be sure to practice them individually before piecing them all together into a cohesive workout. Keep track of each workout as you progress and adapt.

LISTEN TO YOUR BODY

Consult your physician before beginning *Pilates for Athletes* practice. Listen to your body and make changes and modifications accordingly. Pay attention to how you feel from exercise to exercise. Begin slowly and build it each day. Be honest with yourself. Avoid pushing yourself too much or too little. If pain occurs, stop what you're doing completely or use a modification. You should never feel pain in Pilates; you should feel challenged.

Be the master of your own practice and share your discoveries with your teammates, coaches, family and friends. Work to enjoy the flows and look forward to your practice. Feel alive on the mat and boost your athletic expertise. Be excited. Be present. Be a lifelong student.

> You can practice all the flows presented in Chapter 5 of this book with me via online video at **SeanVigueFitness.com/Pilatesforathletesbook**.

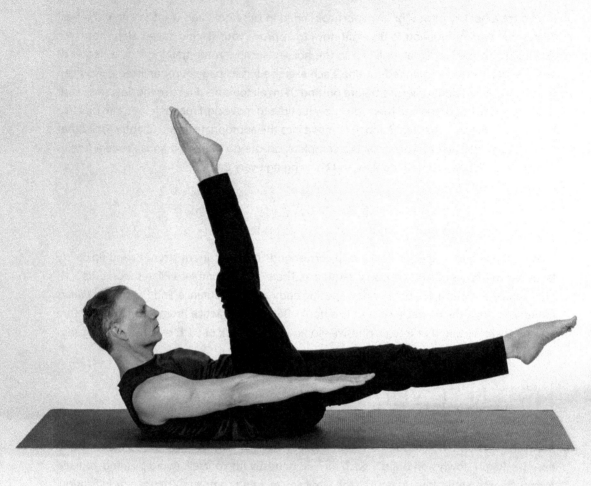

CHAPTER 1

Why Athletes Need Pilates Mat Training

Pilates mat training is a bodyweight-only, total body conditioning program which features an exhaustive list of core centered exercises, sequenced together to elevate your mind, body, spirit and athletic ability. Only a Pilates (or yoga) mat is needed to participate. No weights. No machines. Just you and the mat.

Strictly speaking, there are not many workout programs that can deliver to an athlete the vast amount of benefits that Pilates mat can. It is a lifelong program for the well-rounded athlete to practice, absorb and enjoy. The benefits are almost too exhausting to list, and there is no end to the ways Pilates elevates your health, fitness, movement, speed, strength, control, balance, endurance, breath control, focus, power and flexibility. We'll hit on the big ones a bit later when we get into the classic six principles of Pilates (plus two new ones.)

I don't want to give you a lot of big pep talks in this book because, in my experience, athletes are already motivated and ready to engage in any workout which will make them better, stronger and faster. Athletes are not typically found sitting on a couch talking about the theories of exercise and waiting for an instructor to come by, pick them up and set them moving. If you're an athlete—and you are if you've picked up and gotten this far in the book— you are looking for ways to motivate and inspire yourself through new and effective training techniques which will improve your ability to play and participate in your chosen sports. You want results and you're willing to put in the time and energy to achieve them by any means necessary. If it's going to add strength, speed, precision, control and endurance to your sport, then we're good to go!

When I work with athletes, I find they usually want to get right to the exercises. They always come in with a target in mind. "What stretch is great for tight hamstrings from cycling?" "How do I build a stronger core for tennis forehands?" "How does power yoga improve my explosive speed for football?" Athletes want immediate tools which will help fill in the gaps of their training and show quick improvement for their next practice or game. And there are certainly Pilates exercises to help an athlete up their game on every level, but it's also important that we discuss the big question: Why? Why is Pilates a secret weapon for athletes of all ages and fitness levels? Why is the Pilates mat method a complete training program, all without utilizing any weights, equipment or machines of any kind?

As it happens, Pilates mat was a favorite of the program's founder, Joseph Pilates. The mat approach, i.e. bodyweight-only training, lets you take advantage of the greatest gym you will ever possess: your body. Your body is your vessel for athletic performance, so it pays to create a great relationship with it. With Pilates, the athlete is in possession of a complete conditioning program that fits into even the busiest of schedules.

TOP 10 REASONS WHY ATHLETES *NEED* PILATES MAT TRAINING

1. Pilates constructs a strong, durable, flexible and balanced core.

Joseph Pilates referred to the core as your "powerhouse" and "girdle of strength". It is the center and support of your body. The core is the structural foundation that connects the rest of the body together and develops stability, strength, and control. It begins at the base of the pelvic floor and runs upward to the bottom of the diaphragm, and consists of your abdominals, low back and glutes. Technically speaking, the core is made up of the rectus abdominis (the muscle people mean when they think "abs"), transverse abdominis (the deepest of the abdominal muscles which wraps around your sides and spine), erector spinae (a pair of muscles in your lower back), the internal and external obliques (the muscles located on the sides of your abdomen) and the glutes/bottom/butt (the gluteus maximus, medius, and minimus).

A weak core leaves the athlete open to injuries, compromised endurance and becoming easily fatigued from failing posture. Pilates core exercises train the muscles in your pelvis, lower back, hips, glutes and abdomen to work together, leading to improved balance, stability and body control. Every sport from basketball to tennis to throwing darts depends on force radiating from your center (core) outwards into the limbs.

The core also supports the spine, absorbs shocks in the body and attaches the upper and lower part of the body. If your core is strong, balanced and flexible, your movements will follow suit.

Developing a strong core also helps keeps your posture balanced. Do you catch yourself slouching? Are your shoulders rolled forward right now? Is your low back tight? As an elite (and at all other levels) athlete, your core must be trained to support and balance your body and its everchanging and unpredictable needs.

2. Pilates builds a strong, balanced and resilient body.

Athletes of all ages and fitness levels have been incorporating Pilates into their training for improved overall strength, balance and resistance to injury. This is because it is difficult to find a more comprehensive and effective program than a regular Pilates mat practice. Pilates helps athletes improve their everchanging movement patterns with progressive destabilization, meaning the further you journey into your workouts, the more the exercises will work to challenge and force your body to adapt and improve. Once your body adapts you acquire a higher level of skill.

Each exercise is equally balanced on both sides of the body to counteract the imbalances seen in sports such as tennis, golf or baseball, where the dominant side is favored and strengthened while the other side weakens and atrophies. Pilates works to fix muscular imbalances and bring symmetry to the body, bringing with it optimal physical achievement.

Muscular power and force are essential for peak athletic performance, whether it's slamming your heels down while climbing a grueling hill in cycling, activating your core to swing a baseball bat at a 100 mph fastball, or using your entire body to tackle a fast and elusive 225 lb. running back in football. Pilates teaches to you harness and control the power you need to play well, dominate and win.

3. Pilates improves mobility and ease of movement.

Pilates exercises emphasize healthy, flowing and correct movement. Is your body mobile? How capable are you of moving your body quickly without strain? Are you able to move freely through the day without tightness and discomfort in your body? How well do you move as an athlete? Is your mobility helping or hurting your athletic skill?

How well you move your body through multiple planes of movement determines your athletic success. Pilates training moves your body through every angle and plane of movement while focusing on building strength and flexibility in your core. Having a body which can easily adapt to the unpredictable demands of a sport—quick changes of direction in tennis, explosive speed in hockey, driving to the basket in basketball—will give you a huge edge over your opponents and prolong your career.

4. Pilates improves overall flexibility.

Joseph Pilates once said, "True flexibility can be achieved only when all muscles are uniformly developed." For this reason, Pilates doesn't increase flexibility (defined as the range of motion in a joint or group of joints and moving them through a full range of motion) just based on the popular "hot spots" of the body, such as the hamstrings and low back. Rather, Pilates works through constant flows and movements which stretch, lengthen and expand the whole body. Where many workouts isolate muscles and compress the body and spine, Pilates does just the opposite: every Pilates exercise is designed to lengthen and expand your body through a myriad of flows and angles. It is flowing, dynamic movement which stretches and strengthens the muscles simultaneously. You will smoothly and gracefully flow from one threshold to the next, moving your body with precision and control through as full a range of motion as possible. The challenge is to maintain proper posture, alignment, control and stability while moving through each exercise and the transitions in between.

5. Pilates is a great tool for rehabbing your body during injury and fixing problems associated with muscular imbalance.

Pilates mat practice is low impact on the joints, making it the ideal exercise when rehabbing your body and recovering from an injury. You can also structure your Pilates workouts to your individual needs—there is no one-size-fits-all approach to Pilates. In this book alone, there are over 200 exercises and each one will meet you where you need it to. You are in control of your training, not the exercises. They exist to serve you and your specific physical, mental and conditioning needs.

Remember: with Pilates, the practitioner is responsible for their own rehabilitation. You wouldn't visit a therapist and have them work on you and move your body in all directions while you lay on your back. With Pilates, a patient builds awareness of where their body is in space and how to identify the best movement sequence.

6. Pilates mat only uses your bodyweight, so you can train anywhere and anytime.

Efficient and easily adaptable to your current training program, Pilates can fit into the busiest of schedules. No weights, equipment or machines of any kind means you can rely exclusively on the greatest gym you will ever have: your body.

An athlete needs to train daily to achieve optimum improvement in their body's conditioning and enhance their ability to compete and thrive. The world of Pilates mat is contained in your body, so it can be activated whenever you want or need to train. Whether you are in the gym, at home, on the field, in the locker room or in the mat room, you can access over

200 athletic enhancing exercises in the time it takes to inhale, exhale, roll out your mat (or just train right on the ground, I do it all the time) and bring your body into position. Your workouts can last from 10–60 minutes depending on how much strength, flexibility and focus you need at that moment, and you can train every day, mixing up your workouts so you are consistently hitting new areas.

7. Pilates provides an everchanging, never-ending supply of exercises and sequences to keep you constantly challenged.

Athletes needs to be challenged every day to force their bodies to adapt and improve. Pilates training is a journey of progressive destabilization with every workout. The exercises become more challenging and integrative as you progress, and with each new exercise, you integrate new parts of your body into the movements. Once the exercise becomes too "easy", we add a movement which forces your body to adapt and improve in real time. No matter what the athlete needs, Pilates can supply it.

Even the duration, specific sequence of exercises and focus of the workout (core, flexibility, rehab, strength, back, etc.) can be continually adjusted and changed depending what specifically the solo athlete or team requires. Pilates puts the athlete in control of their training and the workout options are endless.

8. Pilates builds and reinforces proper posture and alignment.

Having proper body alignment—how the head, shoulders, spine, hips, knees and ankles relate and line up with each other—improves your posture and reduces the stress and strain on the spine. Standing, sitting and moving with proper postural alignment will decrease strain on your muscles and ligaments and increase your ability to flow with more efficiency and precision. For athletes, the foundation of control begins with good posture. From this foundation comes the big movements such as jumping, tackling, swinging, throwing, catching and sprinting . . . but if your body is not aligned correctly, these movements will be compromised and weak.

Good posture, working in tandem with a strong core, helps stabilize the body and support the athlete's need for speed, power, rotational force and quick changes of direction. Pilates will help reinforce good posture and alignment during every phase of your sport, no matter how intense or brutal it is.

9. Pilates improves your ability to breathe.

As Joseph Pilates was fond of saying, "Breathing is the first act of life, and the last." Too often, we breathe in a shallow method, draining our energy and focus and crippling our posture. Deep Pilates breathing strengthens the core and lifts our bodies into a strong, aligned posture.

Pilates teaches deep lateral thoracic breathing, which draws the breath upward out of the low belly and bring it into the sides and the low back. This style of breathing drenches the lungs and muscles in oxygen and increases your ability to bring in and process the breath with efficiency. It helps you take advantage of every breath cycle, drawing fresh oxygen into the lungs and squeezing every atom of breath out, filling and emptying the lungs with every breath.

Improving your ability to breathe will drastically increase your athletic performance and abilities. Effective breathing requires thoracic mobility, core strength and a pliable diaphragm for pumping the breath in and out of the lungs. An athlete who is utilizing their full breathing potential will experience increased energy, more blood flow, sharper focus, and improvement when facing stressful and unpredictable situations. Pilates also teaches the athlete how to breathe *into* the movement, which helps the exercises flow smoother through the full range of motion and with more control. Deeper breathing and increased awareness of the breath translates into better form and power with swings, jumps, sprints, changes of directions and throws. Connect your breath with movement and decrease the wear and tear while elevating your ability to move—a win-win-win.

10. Pilates increase your explosive speed and power.

The Pilates combo of deep, expanded breathing, a stronger core, improved flexibility in the entire body, increased strength and efficient movement combine to create a body which can move quicker, faster and with more force behind it. It's pretty straightforward: the looser and more in control you are of your body, the faster your speed and more functional your strength. Whether it means moving quicker with more precision when rolling out for a football pass, maneuvering around the defense en route to the goal in hockey, or planting, jumping and spiking the ball in volleyball with explosive power, Pilates provides the tools to do it.

I am fond of telling athletes to add Pilates to their training before their rival does—the benefits are that powerful and transcend all sports. Every breath you take and every move you make enhances your physical and mental performance, combining to create a deep-rooted love of bettering yourself each and every day. In this, Pilates is a constant and dedicated companion.

Read on to learn the nuts and bolts of what drives a Pilates practice—the eight classic principles of Pilates. You'll also learn why we Pilates instructors, practitioners and aficionados are such a disciplined and methodical group—not only on the mat but in every daily activity.

Oh, and welcome to the lifechanging world of Pilates!

THE EIGHT ESSENTIAL PRINCIPLES OF PILATES

Breath

We talked about breath in the previous section, but it needs to be brought up again (and again and again) to emphasize the life-changing and athletic performance-enhancing qualities it possesses. As I mentioned, Pilates breathing is known as lateral thoracic breathing. This powerful yet efficient way of breathing brings much to the athlete, including more stamina, better posture and the ability to attach the breath effectively to any kind of movement. You can practice this breathing any time of the day from any position. Think of your lungs like any other muscles; they must be continually engaged to become stronger.

Here's how it works: Place your hands on the sides of your body around the rib cage, and breathe in through the nose and out through the mouth. The filters in the nose help purify the air coming in, while exhaling out through the mouth squeezes every drop of breath from the lungs. We aim to squeeze every drop of breath from the lungs every time. Breathe into the rib cage and feel your front, sides and back expand evenly. Feel your upper body expand and lift with the inhale, and let the shoulders sink back and down and the belly button draw into the spine on the exhale. Fill and empty the lungs for maximum lung capacity.

In your Pilates practice, when the going gets tough your ability to breathe will determine your success, precision and stamina. The same applies for your athletic conditioning. Your ability to have a targeted breath focus will determine your effectiveness in practice, games and even into the post-season where injuries and exhaustion can bring us down.

And don't worry if you get dizzy at first—this much oxygen can be intoxicating!

A WORD ON STOMACH VACUUMING (AND ITS BENEFITS)

Practicing the technique known as stomach vacuuming benefits not just your pelvic floor muscles but your core as well. Better yet, it is an exercise you can perform throughout the day no matter where you are. The stomach vacuum activates the transverse abdominis abdominal (the deep layer of muscle behind your rectus abdominis) and affects both your cardiovascular system (by increasing lung strength) and increases the amount of oxygen you can inhale and exhale through your respiratory system.

To practice the stomach vacuum, stand tall and aligned with your hands on your hips. Breathe fully into your lungs, expanding the front, sides and low back. Exhale all the air out of your lungs, totally and completely. Open up your chest and pull your stomach as close as possible to your spine. Hold for a beat and repeat. Give yourself a mental picture of bringing your belly button to the spine.

Repeat for 5–10 reps at a time, remembering to hold yourself upright and tall with an expanding chest. Maintain strong posture throughout. You may also practice vacuuming while seated or on your back. This is an effective move to add to your physical performance arsenal!

Concentration

You probably hear the term "mind/body connection" thrown around a lot, but what does that really mean? In the simplest terms, it means the mind sees it and the body does it—where the mind goes, the body follows. Your mind truly is the boss, and what it says goes.

In Pilates, your mind is the guiding force from exercise to exercise, sequence to sequence, breath to breath. If your mind drifts, your body will tag along.

I also like to use the word "focus" when describing this relationship between the mental and physical. Your focus determines your reality, and regular Pilates practice demands strict and rigorous attention to detail. Without proper focus, I find myself incapable of performing a task, activity, exercise or athletic movement effectively. Trying to accomplish a task without this proper concentration is . . . *frustrating*. I *know* I can do it better, but my lack of focus handicaps my skills.

I believe that when your focus is on point, all Pilates movements flow into one all-powerful principle combining control, purpose, breath, precision, flow, effortlessness and maximum enjoyment. You have to bring all your focus to bear on your movements, both on and off the field. Because no matter where the athlete finds themselves, if there isn't a strong concentration on the present situation, failure is inevitable.

Flow

Flow. What a lovely word—effortless, strong and continuous. Moving continuously while building strength. Without flow, we have exercise chaos.

Pilates flow is a paradox: the more you move, the more energy and endurance you create. It goes against what most people think of a workout—the idea that the more you exercise, the more fatigued you become. Not so with Pilates: as you lock your mind and body into the flow from exercise to exercise, sequence to sequence, breath to breath, you can *feel* your body adapting quickly and in real time.

I'll give an example: in preparing to write this book, I put myself through complete and diverse Pilates exercises daily to understand each and every nuance. With additional practice, my body became hungry for more. My transitions were smoother, my exercises tighter, my breathing deeper and concentration sharper. It's as if I was learning a new language and becoming able to converse freely and effectively without thinking. I began to move from instinct. As my body conquered each new challenge, my connection to my center (core) increased. The deeper that core connection, the deeper the flow.

Pilates teaches athletes to flow effortlessly, creating less wear and tear on the body. This flow will guide the athlete with precision: avoiding hits in football, better follow-through in golf, superior body mechanics in running, and effortless grappling in the martial arts.

Control

Do you have control over yourself? By that I mean, do you *really* have control over your body parts? Are you able to will your body to move however you want? And can you control your thoughts and emotions?

That last question is unexpected, I'm sure. What do thoughts and feelings have to do with physical exercise? As mentioned in the above section on focus, I believe that where the mind goes, the body follows. If your mind is drifting away from your current activity it is impossible to perform at 100 percent, as an elite high-performance athlete should. Pilates teaches and persistently reinforces proper control by giving you so many precise movements to perform that you have no *time* to drift off—it's 100 percent all the time, or nothing. That's the Pilates way. Do it with everything you have . . . and next time will be even better.

Your aim is total mastery of your mind, body and spirit. The athlete must be in control of their emotions and thoughts to stay in the play, in the moment and in the game. It is quite a revelation when you discover how pivotal the power of your mind is in guiding the vast potential of your body. Even when mentally and physically exhausted, you'll still be able to continue playing at an advanced level.

Centering

When a new client steps into my live classes, I always give them "the spiel". The spiel is my verbal introduction to what Pilates is and what they can expect from the class. And the first thing I explain is that Pilates works you from your core outward, like a smoldering fire expanding into all the extremities.

Centering means bringing your focus inward, to the center of your body. As you focus inward, you bring calm to body, mind and spirit. Pilates refers to the center of your torso as the "powerhouse," from which all energy for exercise originates, and having a strong, balanced core will maximize your athletic potential.

The benefits of reinforcing and preserving your core are almost too numerous to count . . . but I'll try: it supports both slow and fast movements; creates a stable core to keep you upright and in proper posture; supports and stabilizes the spine; reduces the risk of injury; reduces low back pain; improves sleep . . . to name just a few!

Precision

It is imperative that we, as Pilates practitioners and athletes, maintain precision and placement through each exercise. Pilates is a very exact science of movement; nothing is by accident. Everything requires tremendous discipline of movement which ultimately leads to mastery.

Precision is a result of clean focus and vivid mental imagery, the will and drive to gain complete mastery over your body. It must be maintained through every exercise, breath, thought and sequence. We also strive to have correct placement of our bodies before beginning each exercise, so proper form is always paramount to our success. Precision also creates a good, steady rhythm which enables our bodies to work honestly and in total control, not using momentum or creating jarring and jerky movements.

What the athlete strives to perfect on the mat will translate to their sport performance. Are you striving to be an average athlete or an elite one? Your dedication to mental and physical precision will answer that question.

Challenge

I've added challenge to this list because, in life, if it doesn't challenge you, it won't change you in a positive way. Pilates—when performed using all the above principles—will be one of the most challenging experiences of your life . . . and the most rewarding. The will to keep striving, keep flowing, keep working and pushing past your thresholds is what breaks barriers, unearths potential, elevates our lives and determines our success in sports, from recreational, high school, college and onto the professional level. Each time you plop yourself on the mat for a Pilates workout, you will be *challenged*. If you aren't, then you simply beef up your workout with the many exercises and flows in this book.

Facing a challenge and accomplishing it lights an inner fire within us which drives us to greater athletic ability. We learn to love and look forward to the challenge, to experience how much we are capable of, to dig deep and reveal our true power and potential. It all begins with the desire to step into the unknown and fight our way through. And that begins with embracing perpetual challenge in our training.

Youth

I am fond of saying "flexibility is youth", and it's true: the looser, more supple and greater range of motion your body possesses, the more you'll find yourself transported back to a time when you rolled out of bed and played all day long. Running, crawling, jumping, biking, fighting and playing sports for hours and hours each day, armed with an unlimited supply of energy and vitality. You never stopped moving, nor felt any of the effects of fatigue and soreness. The next day you sprung out of bed and went at it again until you reluctantly returned home at dusk, covered in grass stains and sweat. Unlimited movement defined your days and taking a "rest day" would have been ridiculous.

The core strength and flexibility training of Pilates will double down on reclaiming the vitality of your youth. Pilates heals, stretches and energizes. You will increase your body's ability to draw in and process oxygen more efficiently and increase the circulation of fresh blood throughout the body and into the muscles and brain. You will train your mind and body to operate on a very high-performance level with no jarring impact on the joints or compression of the spine. You'll feel like *you* again . . . and it will be glorious.

A QUICK OVERVIEW OF PILATES ANATOMY AND ALIGNMENT

We've discussed how your core muscles are at the center of all your strength and movement, that all motion begins in the core. But your core is not just your abdominals, as many people believe, but your entire torso (excluding your arms and legs). It begins at the base of the pelvic floor and runs upward to the bottom of the diaphragm. The core is the deep roots and solid trunk of a tree, one which supports your posture and proper, clean alignment. This group of muscles works together to keep your rib cage, spine, hips, and legs in a neutral position.

The balance that a properly strengthened core brings to the athlete's body will leave it feeling lighter, more balanced, and with increased energy reserves, producing more stamina. The taller and more aligned you are, the more energy you have on the field, court or track.

So let's break down the parts of your core to get a better look and sense of what this center of strength, this powerhouse, really encompasses.

We will also look at the spine, which supports all of our movements—from standing to twisting to running to diving. The athlete must strive to have that perfect marriage of core strength and spinal flexibility for optimum physical performance. Pilates is here to help make that marriage fruitful and successful.

For a visual representation of these muscle groups, see the diagrams on pages 20–22.

Abdominal Muscles

Your **transverse abdominis** runs the deepest of all the abdominal muscles, wrapping around your core. The transverse abdominis works in tandem with your pelvic floor muscles to support the spine and pelvis through what we call intra-abdominal pressure (or IAP). This force is the pressure created within the abdominal cavity. Pilates exercises are designed to work in a smooth, controlled manner specifically to avoid excessive and overloading pressure in the abdominals during movements.

Located underneath your rectus abdominis (the muscle which shows your six pack) and running horizontally across your abdomen, the transverse abdominis is your main activating muscle, working any time you move an arm or a leg. It's also activated when you cough. Go ahead, try coughing. Feel that? You will be activating this muscle when instructed to "pull your belly button into your spine", "scoop your abs" or merely "activate your abs".

The **rectus abdominis** muscle is your "six pack" muscle. The elusive and vaunted "six pack" which sells workout videos, abdominal programs and gym memberships derives from developing a strong and lean rectus abdominis muscle. This muscle emanates on the pubic crest and symphysis pubis, which is the front of pubic bone. It inserts on the side of the xiphoid process, which is at the bottom of the sternum, and on the fifth, sixth, and seventh costal cartilages.

But that's pretty technical, so let me put it this way: it is a pair of long, flat muscles running parallel down the front of your abdomen which work with the sternum pubis to bend the body forward or sideways. They are separated by a midline band of connective tissue called the linea alba. The rectus abdominis also assists with breathing, especially when forcefully exhaling.

The last abdominal muscles are the **external and internal obliques**. They are responsible for any twisting and rotating from our center and are located on the sides of your stomach.

The external oblique muscles are located on the outer surface of the sides of the abdomen, on both sides of the rectus abdominis. They lengthen from the lower ribs to the pelvis. The external oblique muscles on the right side of the body twist the trunk to the left and vice versa. They also assist in core stabilization and support any spinal movement.

The internal oblique muscles are found on both sides of the body, just lateral to the abdomen. It originates from the iliac crest, Inguinal ligament and the Thoracolumbar fascia. The internal obliques help with lateral rotation of the trunk (rotation and twisting), flexion of the trunk (bending forward) and lateral flexion (bending side-to-side) of the trunk. They also assist squeezing breath from the lungs when you need to perform a forced and powerful exhale . . . just as in our Pilates breath.

Back Muscles

Playing a huge part in good posture is the erector spinae muscles which work to maintain an erect and upright spine. They also extend the spine backwards and assists in laterally flexing the spine side-to-side. These muscles are really three muscles: spinalis, longissimus, and iliocostalis. Healthy posture is not possible without strong, flexible and balanced erector spinae muscles.

The multifidus muscle is one of the smallest yet packs a powerful wallop when supporting the spine. A series of muscles that attach to the spinal column, the multifidus muscles work to whisk pressure off the vertebral discs and allow our bodyweight to be uniformly dispersed along the spine. They also work to stabilize and straighten the spine and assist in bending backwards, side-to-side, and rotating to the sides. This amazing muscle also works in tandem with the transverse abdominis and deep pelvic floor muscles to balance and stabilize the low back and pelvis.

These important muscles keep the trunk tall, upright and powerful when performing athletic movements such as running, climbing, jumping, punching, tackling and smashing an overhead tennis or volleyball serve. Pilates has plenty of exercises to keep these muscles healthy, supple and firing on all cylinders.

Glutes

It is important to have strong glutes. If they are not strong enough, the pelvis will not stabilize, and your hamstrings will pick up the slack. As a result, the hamstrings will tighten and send pain and discomfort into the lower back.

Your glutes (the gluteus maximus, gluteus medius and gluteus minimus) must be well-rounded and strong to power the running, climbing, stopping, sprinting, crouching and jumping that are all natural parts of an athlete's routine. They are a key ingredient in your core/powerhouse and they all support each other. If one ingredient is weakened, the whole core apparatus becomes imbalanced, compromised, and finally fails.

Spine

Your spine is composed of 26 separate bony masses, of which 24 are bones called **vertebrae**. The vertebrae are stacked one on top of the other and comprise the central part of the spine running from the base of the skull all the way to the pelvis.

The sacrum sits at the base of the spine and is made up of five fused vertebrae. It forms the back of the pelvis. Located at the bottom of the sacrum is the tailbone (or coccyx) which

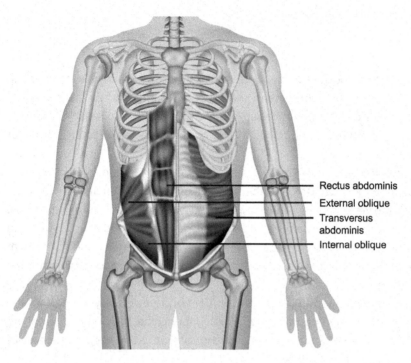

Figure 1. Abdominal Muscles

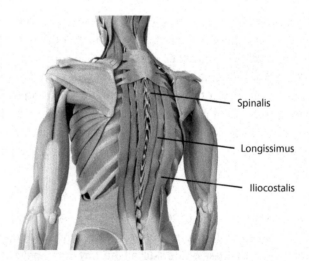

Figure 2. Erector Spinae Muscles of the Back

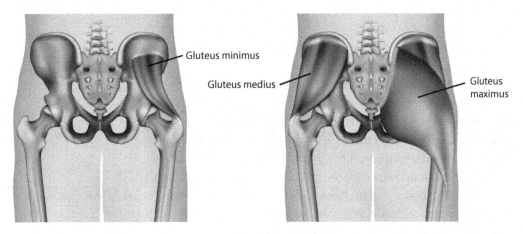

Gluteus minimus

Gluteus medius

Gluteus maximus

Figure 3. Glute Muscles

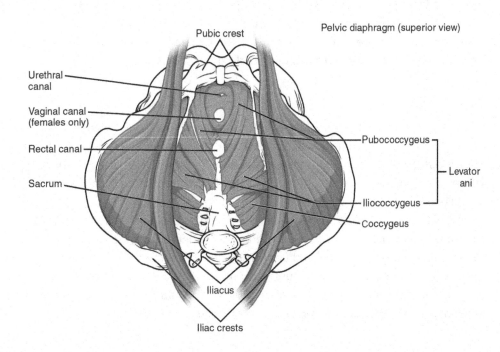

Pubic crest

Pelvic diaphragm (superior view)

Urethral canal

Vaginal canal (females only)

Rectal canal

Sacrum

Pubococcygeus

Iliococcygeus

Coccygeus

Levator ani

Iliacus

Iliac crests

Figure 4. Pelvic Floor Muscles

is made up of four partially fused vertebrae. There are 23 vertebral discs in the spinal column which act as shock absorbers between each bony vertebra, resilient ligaments that hold the vertebrae of the spine together, and cartilaginous joints assisting the mobility of the spine.

The spine is composed of three sections: the **cervical spine**, the **thoracic spine**, and the **lumbar spine**. From the top down, there are seven cervical vertebrae, 12 thoracic vertebrae, and five lumbar vertebrae. The spine acts as a protective barrier for the spinal cord, which is your body's information pathway that delivers signals from the brain to all areas of the body. The healthier your spine, the more efficiently the brain and body send signals back and forth and communicate. This is essential for a strong mind/body connection and enables your body to move as efficiently and precisely as possible, with the brain as the guide. Athletes must make split second decisions and move their bodies quickly and fluidly for matchless physical performance.

Pilates has become an exercise program recommended by many healthcare professionals for athletes with certain spine conditions which inhibit strong movement patterns, as well as for injury prevention and the overall fitness benefits it offers, specifically because of how Pilates works to maintain a healthy, pliable and mobile spine.

Cervical

Thoracic

Lumbar

Sacrum

Coccyx

Pelvic Floor

Pilates training also activates your pelvic floor muscles which are comprised of the muscle fibers of the levator ani, the coccygeus muscle, and the surrounding connective tissues which encompass the area underneath the pelvis. These muscles stretch like a strong and flexible trampoline from the tailbone to the pubic bone (going front to back) and from one of your sitting bones to the other sitting bone (side to side).

It is essential you keep your pelvic muscles strong, as they protect and support the muscle function of areas including the bowels, uterus, vagina and bladder, as well as provide support for the spine and keep the anal and urinary sphincters healthy and functioning. (To feel your pelvic floor at work, activate the muscle you use to stop the flow of urine when urinating.) They also help maintain appropriate intra-abdominal pressure and help facilitate childbirth by helping guide the baby during the descent and through the pelvic girdle.

You will hear the term "C-Curve" bandied about frequently in this book, and for good reason. The C-Curve refers to the shape the spine needs to be in when performing exercises requiring a smooth, rolling motion of the spine; i.e. the roll up, roll over and rolling like a ball. In these movements, the spine is rounded and flexed—including the lumbar spine, which is usually straight—creating an arc similar to the letter "C" which enables it to roll like a wheel from top to bottom. Your chin is tucked and abs scooped to complete the fluid flow. Shoot for an even curvature throughout the spine for the smoothest, healthiest spinal roll.

Pilates engages and enhances spinal flexion (bending and lifting forward), spinal extension (bending and lifting backwards with length) and spinal rotation (rotating right and left). You will have many chances to practice your flexion, extensions and rotations with the plethora of exercises contained in this book, as Pilates will help you flex, twist, extend, and rotate your spine efficiently in every direction in a healthy and controlled manner.

To quote Joseph Pilates: "If your spine is inflexibly stiff at 30, you are old. If it is completely flexible at 60, you are young."

THE PILATES STANCE

The Pilates Stance is a position used in many Pilates exercises to engage the legs and deepen the engagement of the core. In this position, the legs are extended, squeezed together, toes pointed and heels pressing into one another (think of tightly zipping up the legs with a zipper). This shape is also called the Pilates V shape.

The Pilates Stance sets up the practitioner into a neutral position. It is a position to adhere to when getting ready to exercise—it is *not* a standalone exercise. Rather, it is meant to bring focus to the body's alignment and location during all Pilates exercises. It is wonderful for engaging your legs, glutes, hips, core, quads, hamstrings and feet and will help you perform all the exercises more effectively and with greater balance and power.

Now that we've had an overview of the primary anatomy of Pilates, let's take a look at how best to optimize one's Pilates practice—and how we can make it happen.

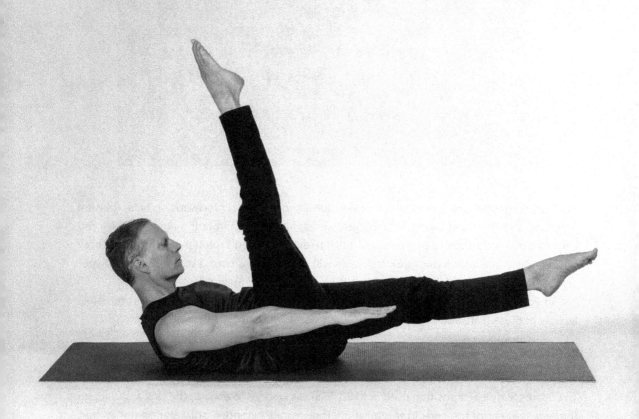

CHAPTER 2

How to Build Your Own Pilates Practice

As an athlete, you want to get the most bang for your buck when it comes to training. You're not going to put in all the time and energy needed to learn the Pilates mat method only to set the bar low and aim for a subpar workout experience, are you?

Pilates demands precision—and is here to drench your mind and body with unstoppable benefits which enhance your athletic abilities. We are upgrading all your resources with the exercises, flows and training logs in this book and that means avoiding anything that might sabotage or diminish your unlimited potential.

With that in mind, here are some tips to help deliver the best possible Pilates training experience wherever and whenever you decide to drop onto your mat and elevate your sports skills.

No Music

This goes against the prevailing opinion that adding your favorite heart-raising, fist pumping playlist to your workouts will produce more energy, increase adrenaline and get you better results—not to mention boost the body's levels of serotonin and dopamine. And sure, when I do strength training or hit the pavement for a run, you bet that I load up my iPod (yes, I still use one) with plenty of high energy songs (lots of Mötley Crüe, too) to give me that extra kick in the butt to train with power and psych me up to sling and lift progressively heavier weights.

Pilates training is *different*. Music is a *distraction* in Pilates. When honing your Pilates exercises, it is paramount that your ears are filled with the exhilarating sounds of only your breath (and an occasional grunt). Breath and movement bind together in Pilates to create the most fluid and precise fitness experience possible, all without any other distracting sounds or beats.

Pilates exercises also have a distinct and steady rhythm that intrusive music can disrupt and shatter. Train only with the natural sounds of your physical exertion and you will find out what you are really made of. Spend some good, quality time with yourself.

Begin with a Dynamic Stretch Warm-up

The flows in this book have built-in exercises and movements to get the blood flowing and the body limber, but the addition of dynamic stretching (active movements which send the muscles and joints through a controlled full range of motion) will increase blood flow, body awareness and warm up the body before jumping full force into your Pilates workout. Dynamic stretches are valuable for athletes who need to perform a lot of jumping and running, as in basketball, football, soccer and volleyball. They enhance your cardiovascular performance and reduce the risk of injury.

> To do a dynamic stretch warm-up with Sean, visit **SeanVigueFitness.com/PilatesforAthletesBook**.

Train with Your Teammates/Coaches

As a Pilates practitioner, the only people you should NOT share Pilates with . . . are your rivals. Why share this secret weapon for peak athletic performance with your opponents?

But by all means, share your knowledge of Pilates mat training with your teammates and coaches! Just by going through the flows and training logs in this book, you will see a performance increase across the board. Set up times to practice together, build a Pilates program within your team—your teammates deserve to experience the power of Pilates training for themselves, and you're the one to lead them to elevated athletic prowess. For your coaches, not only will they experience the benefits but Pilates, it will also strengthen the bonds of the team as a whole as you all struggle and succeed together with Pilates the same way you do during practice and on game day.

Practice Pilates together as your pre-practice/game warm-up, as a solo workout for a core/energy boost, or as an off-day session when your body needs to change things up and have an active rest. Pilates meets you where you are at any given moment. Athletes appreciate and need this high level of efficiency and adaptability.

Plan Around Mealtimes

Food in the belly and Pilates usually don't mix. The core-centered intensity of Pilates doesn't play nice when it encounters food competing for stomach space. Stomach cramps, abdominal pain and even vomiting can happen when your stomach is too full during exercise. Trying to pull that belly button up and in while being blocked by your last meal is neither comfortable nor enticing. Training too soon after eating also diverts blood and energy away from the digestion process and into the muscles, causing uneasy sensations such as gas, cramping and bloating. Experiencing these discomforts will make you just want to hang it up for the day and head home for a nap, and now you've missed your workout.

Plan to eat at least an hour before your Pilates session (two hours if you're having a big meal). A full meal of protein, fat, and fruits or vegetables eaten two hours before your Pilates workout will give you plenty of time to digest. Protein and fat burn gradually and digest slowly, so by the time you begin Pilates you will have the stamina to carry you through the workout. If you must eat one hour before, try oatmeal (my favorite pre-Pilates snack), nuts, yogurt or a protein bar.

These are merely my personal suggestions, so find what food/meals work best to give you consistent energy without feeling bloated and constricted in your movements.

Take Days Off

As enjoyable, beneficial and even intoxicating as the world of Pilates is, it's important to take days off now and then to recharge and recover. I say this because Pilates can become very addictive. Every session elevates your mind, body and mood. You feel better and uplifted after each session. You have more energy after each session—you walk taller, with better alignment. With so many positive benefits, it is easy to overdo your practice without even realizing it. As an athlete, you owe it to yourself to train smart with Pilates and find balance.

Unplug

Pilates training gives you a golden opportunity to escape the many distractions of modern society and return to your true nature. All those tiny little screens are frying our eyeballs and severing our attention span. Your Pilates workouts are a chance to spend time with your thoughts, breath, dreams, goals and whatever else the world has distracted you from. Take advantage of this private time with yourself and emerge refreshed, focused and calm.

Practice Outside

This goes along with the above tip on unplugging. I'm a big fan of taking all my workouts outside, not just Pilates—temperature-controlled buildings and shiny weight rooms leave me wanting and uninspired, while getting outside enhances the mood. Sunshine, fresh air and the natural elements are very inspiring and healing. (In fact, I wrote most of this book while sitting outside on my deck surrounded by trees, elk, blue skies, my son Dane and my dog Addie.)

Practicing your Pilates outside brings you directly in touch with nature and yourself. Unlike at the gym, there are no people wanting to chat right in the middle of your Pilates 100, no fluorescent lights blinding the eyes or members stepping over you to use the squat rack. So step outside with Pilates for some vitamin D and invigoration. Don't forget to grab your teammates!

Sleep More

Lack of sleep will make your Pilates exercises and flows very sloppy. I know from experience: when I'm drowsy and try to launch into a Pilates routine (or teach one), my cues, rhythm and flow are off. It feels like sleepwalking.

If your Pilates session is not coming together, then it's coming apart. A good night's sleep makes you energized and alert while improving your cognitive function and focus. Your mood will also be heightened, creating a more positive Pilates experience. More athletic performance-enhancing benefits of sufficient sleep include staying at a healthy weight, lower risk for diabetes and heart disease, reduced inflammation and increased reaction times. For overall health, sufficient sleep is always a good idea.

Hydrate Properly

Not getting enough sleep is about as detrimental to your athletic performance as not taking in an ample amount of fresh, clean water on a daily basis. It's hard to argue against staying hydrated when our bodies are 60% water (with blood a whopping 90% water).

Are you ready to hear the many benefits of switching off soft drinks and making water your main squeeze? Drinking water (6–8 glasses per day) lubricates the joints, carries oxygen throughout the body, regulates body temperature, boosts your athletic and physical performance abilities, and supports healthy digestion.

It is not recommended that you drink a lot of water *before* doing your Pilates workout as the extra amount of liquid sloshing in your belly might interfere with your core work and engagement. Have a few sips before beginning and maybe take a quick break during to have a couple more. Your body will let you know if it's too much, too little, or just right.

Keep a Pilates Training Journal

Planning, making notes and reviewing progress in your daily Pilates training will help clarify and focus your fitness goals. No two workouts are the same, so it's important to track your progress and work on areas which need help.

What You Need to Practice

Pilates demands unrestricted movement, so wear loose, comfortable clothes. Yoga pants, leggings, sweatpants and shorts work great when paired with tank tops, T-shirts and fitted, stretchy tops. If it doesn't restrict your range of motion, it's a keeper.

You'll also need a Pilates or yoga mat. Pilates mats have a little more support and feel "squishy"; this extra thickness is needed for supporting and cushioning the spine when performing rolling exercises such as rolling like a ball, roll ups and roll overs. Yoga mats also work very well if you're okay with a little less softness. Roll either one out, smooth out the edges, and prepare to blast off!

Other than adding your body, that's it! No weights or machines required. You're using the greatest gym ever—your body—to its full advantage.

Your *Pilates for Athletes* studies begin in the next chapter, where I'll be providing you with the tools to move: the warm-ups and exercises.

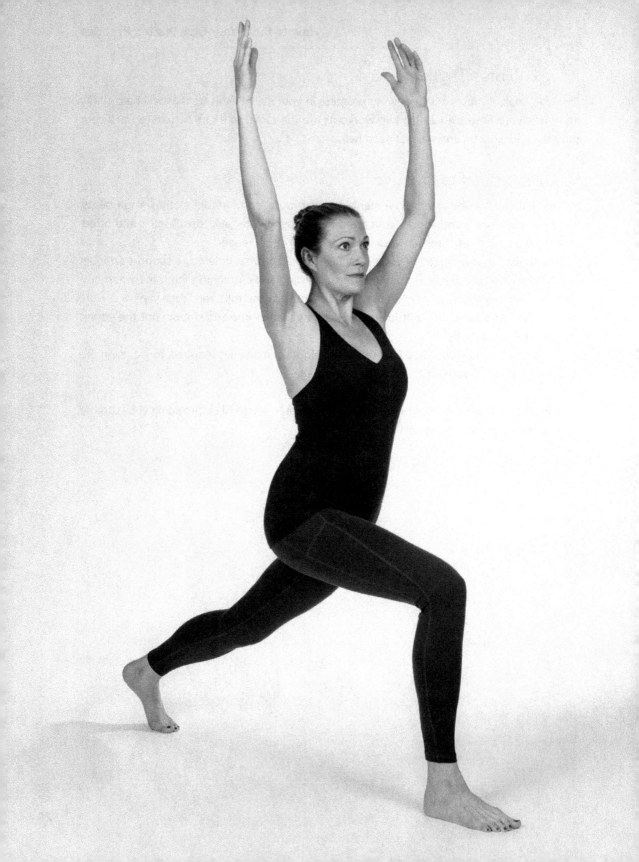

CHAPTER 3

Warm-ups

I t's always a great idea to warm up the body before diving into a full Pilates workout. Warming up raises your heart rate, drives fresh oxygen through the body, increases blood flow (which heats up the muscles and makes them more pliable), and sharpens your focus.

You want to make sure you're firing on all cylinders each and every time you set aside time for your Pilates practice. In fact, your warm-up may be the most important aspect of your overall training because it sets the tone and brings all your senses online to focus on the task at hand. Let's commit to making every Pilates session a huge success—one which will keep us coming back for more.

These warm-up exercises and stretches are designed to lead you into your practice. I've also added a few yoga poses to amp up your focus and flexibility. Be sure to practice classic Pilates breathing throughout by inhaling through the nose and exhaling out the mouth. Breath builds your foundation.

I want to add that walking is a phenomenal warm-up and a great overall activity for building health, wellness and clarity. Before I begin my Pilates workout, you'll find me walking outside around my neighborhood to clear my head and bring a steady flow of blood to my muscles. As Ralph Waldo Emerson said, "Walking has the best value as gymnastics of the mind."

◼ MOUNTAIN

Mountain is a great beginning stance that focuses on proper posture, alignment and breath.

1. Bring your feet hip-width apart with the toes pointed forward. Keep a little softness in the knees and let your quads lengthen your legs.

2. Roll your shoulders back and down, bringing your arms to your sides. Tuck in your chin as if you're holding an orange between the chin and the chest. Relax your jaw and focus on your breath.

3. Reach your fingers towards the floor and relax your stare at a fixed point.

4. On each exhale, draw your belly button into your spine, creating a contraction in the abdominals and squeezing every drop of breath from the lungs. Inhale and let the breath fill your front, sides and low back.

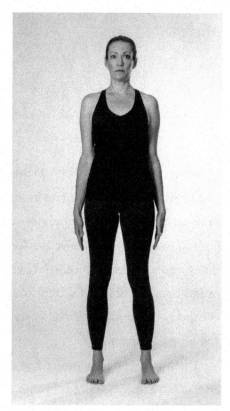

Key Points

- Mountain is the perfect starting point to set up your focus for what is to come. Your time is precious and you want to maximize your workouts. With a clear, strong focus, you increase your capacity for success.

- This pose exhibits many of the Pilates postural themes, including engaging the abdominals with each exhale, keeping the shoulders back and down, the chin slightly tucked to keep a nice line down the back, and using the breath to delve deeper into your body.

Variation

Backbend:

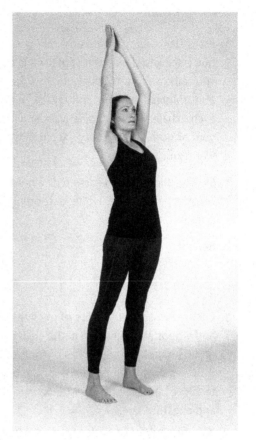

1. From Mountain pose, extend the arms overhead with an inhale and back with the exhale.

2. Try bringing your arms behind your ears while sinking your shoulders down and back. Your fingertips should be softly touching. Tuck your tailbone under your body.

3. Inhale, extend your arms skyward and exhale, letting your arms continue traveling back.

4. Practice for 5–10 seep breaths, in the nose and out the nose.

Key Points

- Backbends are essential for expanding the breath, preventing the "rolling shoulders" forward syndrome which kills our posture, and stretching the abdominals and back to encourage blood flow.

- They also decrease anxiety and stress by broadening the front of the body, including opening the chest, and by extension the heart.

- It's a wonderful way to establish a strong focus and saturation of breath.

Variation

Cactus Arms:

1. From Backbend, exhale and pull your arms out, back and down as if someone is pulling your elbows together behind you. Pull your abdominals into your spine (flex them) on each exhale. We want to activate and include your abdominals in every exercise, even the warm-up.

2. Slowly slide your elbows down for 2–3 breaths and inhale while extending your arms into Backbend.

3. Repeat 5–10 times.

Key Points

- Cactus Arms are a favorite of my live classes and videos. When I teach it, the class usually groans happily in unison as a result of how it opens up the front of the body, relieves tension, and aligns the neck, shoulders and chest.

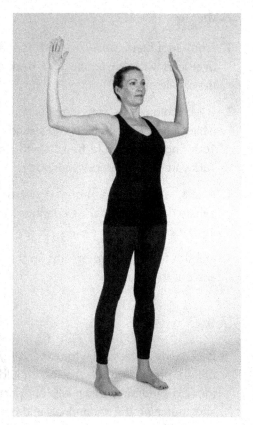

- Your breathing expands as the mind/body marriage takes hold. Remember that our success in training is dependent on how we enter into the practice.

MUDRA

Mudra means "seal" or "closure" in Sanskrit and for our purposes is represented as a finger bind.

1. Exhale and draw your arms behind you and lace your fingers together while dropping your shoulders back and down, opening up the chest.

2. Inhale while lifting your shoulders up slightly and exhale while tugging your hands towards the floor. You may also bring your palms together to increase the stretch in the forearms. Hold for 5–10 breaths.

Key Points

- This pose is a wonderful way to pump more oxygen into your body and align your posture. I use this pose when teaching and filming Power Yoga routines.
- It's a great stimulus for the organs, abdominals and low back.

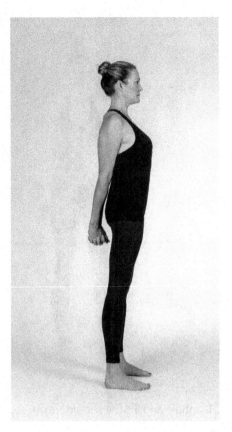

■ SHOULDER ROLLS

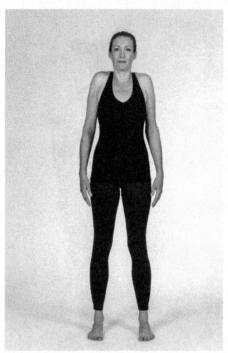 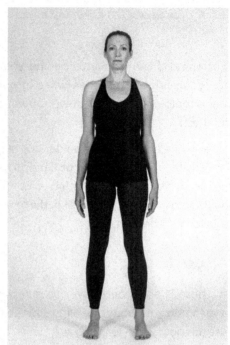

1. Inhale and lift the shoulders up.

2. Exhale and release them down and back. You should feel them sliding down your back. Repeat 5–10 times.

Key Points

- Shoulder rolls are a smooth way to incorporate alignment and postural training into your life with minimal distraction. They can be done anywhere and anytime to great effect.

- Your shoulders will thank you as more blood flow is pumped through these essential muscles.

SIDE BENDS

1. Inhale and reach your right arm straight towards the ceiling.

2. Exhale and bend to the left, leading with your core. Allow your left arm to slide down the side. Repeat 5 times on each side.

Key Points

- These bends lengthen and bring relief to the abdominals, hips and thighs.

- Side bends stretch the muscles between the ribs (intercostals). Tight intercostals cause neck and shoulder tension but stretching them out will open the ribcage and lungs, increasing breath capacity.

- Side bends also stretch the digestive organs which helps digestion and metabolism.

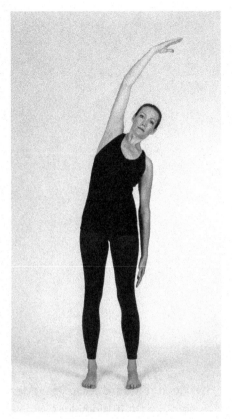

ARM CIRCLES

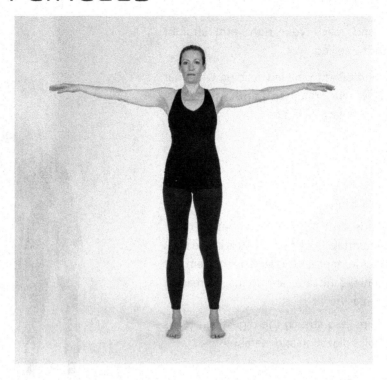

1. Extend your arms out to your sides and circle them forward, relaxing them down. Breathe normally. Do 10 repetitions.

2. Reverse and do 10 more repetitions backwards.

Key Points

- It's important that you don't let your shoulders creep up and forward. Sink them back and down while circling.

- Arm circles bring a lot of fresh blood and heat to the shoulders helping with mobility of movement.

FLOP DOWNS

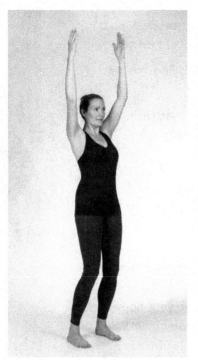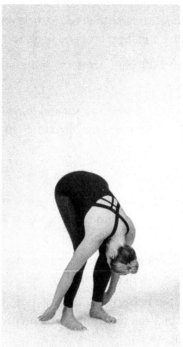

1. Inhale, raising your arms overhead and back. Bend the knees slightly and exhale, swinging your arms downward while increasing the bend in your knees.

2. Inhale, stand tall again, and repeat. Do 5–10 repetitions.

Key Points

- Flop downs stretch the spine, back, hamstrings and calves while activating the core on the upswing.
- The fast, controlled motion increases energy levels, oxygen to the brain and breath control efficiency.
- Your legs will also engage to help keep the movement smooth and controlled.

CHAIR POSE

1. From Mountain pose (page 32, exhale and press back, placing the emphasis in the glutes and heels and out of the knees.

2. Inhale and lift your arms tall without moving the rest of your body.

3. Exhale and keep sinking back and down. On each exhale, give the abdominals a squeeze. Hold for 5–10 breaths.

Key Points

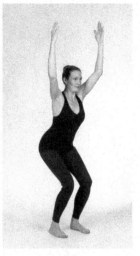

- Chair pose builds strength in the glutes, core, thighs, calves and ankles while increasing focus power. It also adds flexibility to the shins and Achilles tendons.

- Chair really elevates the heart rate and builds heat in the body quickly—the perfect warm-up move.

- Increase the balance of Chair by rising onto your tippy-toes. Keep your eyes fixed on a set point to improve balance and focus.

- Another add-on is to incorporate a twist. Do 10 repetitions total and hold each for 3 breaths.

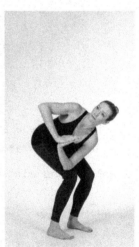

LUNGE

I love lunges of all kinds, but it's necessary to work on the foundation to ensure the best possible form.

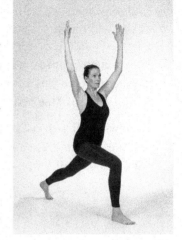

1. Step your right foot forward so your knee is above your ankle. Extend the back leg by pressing the heel towards the floor. You may also bring that knee onto the mat.

2. Keeping your fingers on the mat, inhale and lift your arms up and back, exhale, sinking down into your legs. Do 5–10 breaths on each side.

Key Points

- Lunges build powerful core stability and flexibility while increasing balance.

- Lunges heat up your legs and glutes and helps to cultivate a strong focus on the moment.

Add-on

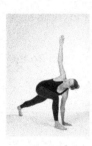

Lunge Twist: Exhale and place your hand on the floor. Inhale and reach your other arm to the sky. Inhale and rotate, drawing your upper shoulder back. Hold for 5–10 breaths on each side.

FORWARD FOLD

Decompressing the spine relieves tension on the spinal discs, releasing them and taking pressure off the nerves and spine. Relieving this tension encourages water, oxygen and nutrients to flow into the discs.

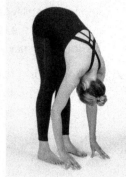

1. From Mountain pose (page 32), exhale, tuck your chin and fold forward from the hips, keeping softness in the knees. Lead with the top (crown) of the head.

2. Sink lower with each exhale and rock your weight into the tips of your toes for a deeper stretch. Allow your legs and spine to help stabilize the pose.

Key Points

- The Sanskrit translation of this movement is "intense stretch pose", and that's about right. Forward Fold stretches the back, hamstrings, calves, shoulders, neck and glutes.

- Dropping your head below your heart is called an "inversion" in yoga and works to calm the mind, relieve headaches, help insomnia and ease anxiety. Avoid rounding the back.

- Use caution when folding. Place your hands on your legs for more support and come back to Mountain pose if you feel dizzy, lightheaded or uncomfortable.

- These folds help create a concentrated focus due to oxygen-rich blood flowing into the brain and head.

Add-ons

Wide-Legged Forward Fold: Space the feet wider for a deeper neck and spine stretch. Modify by placing your hands on your legs for support. Breathe deep and allow your heart rate to come under your control.

Walking Forward Fold: Add a nice stroll with a twist to increase blood flow, flexibility and low back pliability.

Mudra Forward Fold (Regular and Wide Legged): Bind your hands behind you, inhaling while lifting them skyward and exhaling while driving the crown of the head towards the ground. Engage your core to keep you lifted, as your hands are now unavailable for ground support.

DOWNWARD FACING DOG

This pose is the basis not only of my Power Yoga routines but also all other fitness disciplines I practice. All movements are easily accessible from Down Dog.

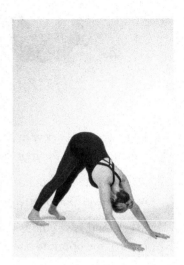

1. From Forward Fold (page 42), walk the hands forward until your body is in an upside-down "V" shape with your hands in front of your shoulders and feet behind the hips.

2. Spread your fingers wide to create a nice foundational base and draw weight off the wrists. Bring your hands shoulders-width and feet hip-width apart.

3. Exhale and sink back towards your heels, bringing them closer to the ground. Relax the shoulders and allow them to pull away from each other creating a nice stretch and allowing blood to flow in the upper back. Keep the chin tucked slightly and draw your nose towards the knees, tailbone up, heels down.

Key Points

- Down Dog is a stretch which drenches the body with energy and rejuvenates the mind. It stretches the shoulders, hamstrings, calves, back, spine and glutes . . . and it feels really good the deeper you delve into the pose.

- The inversion factor in Down Dog also has a calming effect as fresh blood is drawn into the head and brain, helping to center the mind and thoughts.

Add-ons

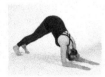

Dolphin: Go further with the Dolphin pose. From Downward Facing Dog, place your forearms on the mat and continue bringing your upper body towards your legs and sinking the heels down. This variation will add extra flexibility and stretch to your arms, shoulders, back and hamstrings

WINDSHIELD WIPERS

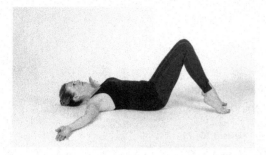 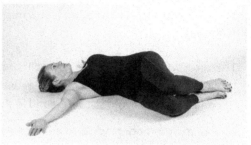

1. Begin on your back with your knees pulled into your chest using your hands. This is also a fantastic stretch for your low back and knees.

2. Place your toes on the ground with an inhale while extending your arms out to the sides or overhead for a deeper shoulder and back stretch.

3. Exhale and lower the legs to your side, keeping the knees bent and turning the upper body in the opposite direction. Turn your head to face opposite, too.

4. Inhale, bring the legs back to center and continue to the other side. Repeat 10 times.

Key Points

- Windshield Wipers are equally effective as a warm-up and cool down as they stretch your back and glutes and hydrate the discs. It is one of the best feeling stretches around; I have yet to find someone who disagrees.

- This is a great move to stretch and realign the spine. Many people experience cavitation (adjustments) during the stretch.

- The twisting motion also delivers more blood to the digestive organs, improving the function of your digestive system.

■ TOE TOUCHES

Let's turn our attention to the abdominals.

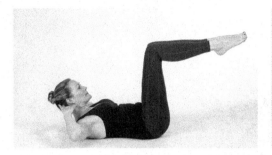 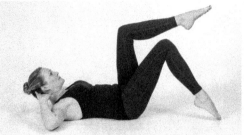

1. Lie on your back and place your fingertips to the outside of the back of the head. Bring your legs to tabletop position with your feet extended directly in front of your knees. Sink your lower back into the mat (imprinting).

2. Exhale and bring your head, neck and shoulders off the ground. Hold this upper body position.

3. Inhale while lowering the right leg (keeping the knee at 90 degrees) until your toes brush the ground.

4. Exhale and return to tabletop position. Alternate 5–10 times on each leg.

Key Points

- We get a wonderful intro into "core stability" with this simple yet challenging exercise. As the legs are moving up and down, our core is keeping the rest of our body stable. Stability against movement: your core is the anchor which retains the solid foundation of each exercise.

- I teach this exercise as a warm-up, but with a slow, steady rhythm it can become very challenging. In fact, you will find that every Pilates exercise is much more rewarding when the tempo is decreased, forcing our muscles to work harder to maintain good form and breath. I recommend studying and mastering all the exercises in the book—and that includes bringing down the tempo and digging deeper into your physical and mental threshold.

- For an added contraction in the abdominals, lift your chest upward when the knee returns to tabletop position.

Add-on

Double Toe Touches: Increase the level of core stability challenge by lowering and raising both legs together. Maintain the imprint of your lower back into the ground.

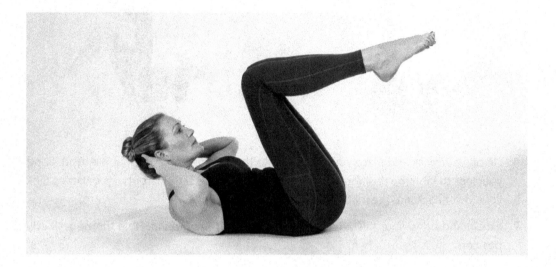

CHEST LIFT

This exercise is commonly called a "crunch" but there's more to it than meets the eye.

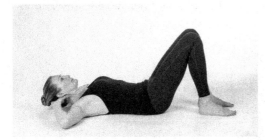 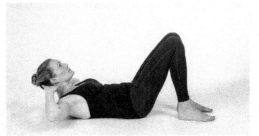

1. Lying on your back, place your feet flat on the floor so that your heels are under your knees. Your fingers are in the same position as Toe Touches (page 45).

2. Exhale and lift your chest towards your knees using the abdominals. You should be peeling your spine off the mat, which we will do in a lot of Pilates exercises.

3. Inhale and slowly return to the starting position, massaging your spine into the mat. Repeat 5–10 times.

Key Points

- Let your elbows stay pointed outward to avoid pulling on the back of the head. You want to have length in the back of the neck (keeping the natural curve) and the chin slightly tucked. I teach this exercise as a warm-up, but with a slow, steady rhythm it can become very challenging. In fact, you will find that every Pilates exercise is much more rewarding when the tempo is decreased, forcing our muscles to work harder to maintain good form and breath. I recommend studying and mastering all the exercises in the book—and that includes bringing down the tempo and digging deeper into your physical and mental threshold.

- It's helpful to have a breath rhythm for this exercise, to set the tone for a successful and un-hurried workout. It's quality over quantity in Pilates. Try exhaling up for four counts, holding on the top for two, and releasing to starting position with four counts. Like a song, Pilates has a consistent rhythm from beginning to end. Set it early in the workout for maximum success and challenge.

- Peel your spine off the mat vertebra by vertebra on the contraction (upward lift) and imprint it vertebra by vertebra on the stretch (downward movement). This precise motion improves spinal flexibility, control and function while massaging the muscles of the back.

Add-on

Chest Lift with Double Toe Touch: Combine these two exercises into a powerful move which engages the abdominals and lower back. Inhale and lower the upper and lower body toward the floor, brush the toes, exhale, and bring the chest and knees together. Repeat 10–20 times.

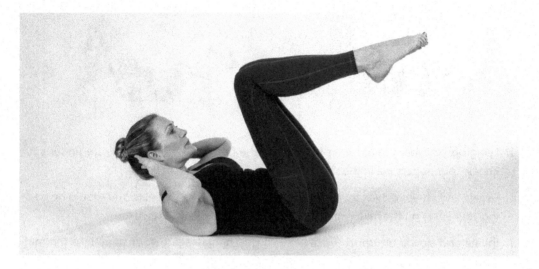

CHAPTER 4

Classic Pilates Mat Exercises

t's time to dive into your Pilates practice. I've put together the original 34 classic Pilates mat exercises to get you on the mat and moving right now. This list includes full descriptions with pictures and key points to ensure you have all the study materials you need to properly perform, practice, and master your Pilates training.

In addition to the classic mat exercises, I've included modifications and add-ons for each exercise. Depending on your skill level, you may choose to begin practicing and mastering the modifications, honing the original exercises before moving on to the add-ons.

The add-ons increase the challenge and difficulty level of each exercise by incorporating more core stability, movement, focus, flexibility and strength. I have added an "Intensity Meter", and so each add-on is listed in order of difficulty (Level 1, Level 2, Level 3, and occasionally the dreaded Master), giving you a clear ladder of progression. As your mind and body build, so do your exercises and flows. Remember: Pilates always meets you where you are.

PILATES 100

AREAS TARGETED: Core, shoulders, adductors and quads

  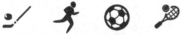

This exercise signals the official start of your Pilates workout—and we're starting with a bang that puts your muscles on notice!

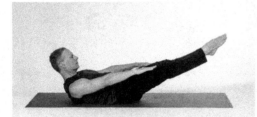 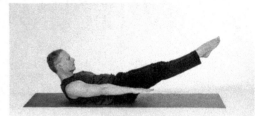

1. Lie on your back, draw your legs to tabletop position and peel the head and shoulder off the mat while raising your arms to the sides. Make sure your low back is imprinted against the mat.

2. Extend the legs and zip them up into Pilates stance (page 23) with the heels together and feet pointed. Deepen the pull of your abdominals to prepare for the incoming movement.

3. While breathing in for 5 counts and out for 5, pump the arms up and down together about 4–6 inches while sinking the shoulders down and back and expanding the chest. Keep the abdominals pulling into the spine on the exhales. The pumping of the arms is in unison with your breath and will last for 100 counts—hence the name of the exercise.

Key Points

- The Pilates 100 is a beautiful demonstration of core stability in action. The core must work extra hard to stabilize the body against the vigorous movement of the arms. Focus on using your center as an anchor against those pumping arms. You can increase the difficulty by lowering your legs closer to the floor, making your core work harder.

- Keep the chin tucked down towards the chest with enough space in between for a small apple. You will feel a nice stretch in the back of your neck and avoid any undue strain. You may also keep your head on the floor (or use a pillow or rolled up towel) if the strain of lifting your head off the floor is too much. (This applies for *all* the exercises in this book.)

- All the pumping married with the staccato breaths saturates your muscles with oxygen and strengthens the lungs.

Add-ons

LEVEL 1

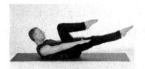

Single Leg Stretch 100: This is an addition to the Single Leg Stretch exercise which you'll learn shortly in the classic 40. Keeping the 100 arm position, draw your right knee in at a 90 degree angle and extend your left leg 45 degrees off the ground or lower (as long as the lower back stays flat). The chin is tucked the same way as the 100 as you inhale for 5 while you pump your arms 4–6 inches and switch your legs in a controlled, smooth movement. Exhale for 5, continuing to pump the arms and return to the starting position. Repeat for 100 breaths. Force the muscles to strengthen with movement and constant disruption.

LEVEL 2

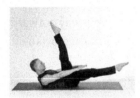

Scissors 100: From Single Leg Stretch 100, simply extend the legs and point the feet. Now you're in a position for the Scissors, which adds more weight and inertia to the movements. Scissor the legs with the constant 5 breaths in and 5 breaths out, all while pumping the arms in a controlled manner. Repeat for 100 breaths. The calibration of the movement between the arms and legs takes practice; Pilates has a lot of moving parts which must synchronize in order for the flow to ignite. Just remember that practice makes the master. When you feel confident with the precision of this exercise, it's time to move on.

LEVEL 3:

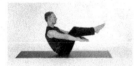

Boat 100: Pop your body up to Boat position. Boat is a classic yoga pose and one which is going to ramp up the core stability, balance and intensity of the 100 exercise, in addition to strengthening the hip flexors which attach the inner thigh bones to the front of the spine. From a seated position, bring your legs to tabletop position (you can also extend your legs to full boat pose, which is brutal) sitting on your sit bones and tailbone. Keep the same chin and arm position as the standard 100 as you once again pump the arms 4–6 inches, palms down and to the precise rhythm of 5 counts in and 5 counts out, in the nose and out the mouth for 100 pulses. It's always in the nose and out the mouth in Pilates; we perform so much better and more efficiently with a constant reinforcement of deep, focused breaths.

You will find the core stability to be rather severe in this pose due to the extra balance adding to the disruption of the core. Just holding Boat is demanding and with the glorious intrusion of the pumping arms, it forces your body and mind to dig deeper and maintain the movement without falling over. You may also extend your legs out on the 5-count inhale and draw them back to Boat with the 5-count exhale.

MASTER

Arms Overhead 100: Now we come to the final variation in the 100 series. We could almost base an entire workout on just this progression of exercises; they are such a dynamic demonstration of discovering, building and putting into practice the eight principles of Pilates listed in Chapter 1. Movement which progressively builds on itself develops the body naturally with very minimal side effects to hinder our practice. That is why this exercise is listed at "Master" intensity level. It enables you to work your way up and master not only the exercise but the movement. Your goal as an athlete is to always perform better, move better, react faster.

Lying on your back, extend the arms overhead and the legs extended in Pilates stance. Imprint your low back into the mat with a strong pelvic tilt. Pump your arms up and down palms up with the 5 count in and 5 count out. Your core will explode in all directions as it works overtime to anchor the body against the weight of the extended arms and legs. Repeat 100 times.

You may also direct the legs as in Single Leg Stretch or the Scissors. Work your way outward from the core and experience your body strengthening in real time towards effortless movement on the field, court and snow hill.

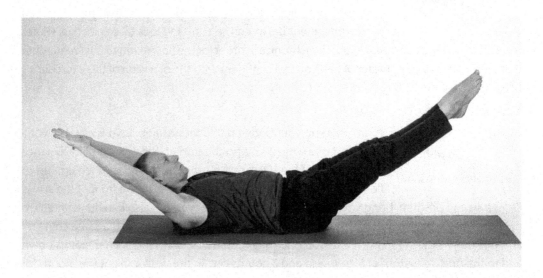

THE ROLL UP

AREAS TARGETED: Core, spine and legs

This exercise forces you to get to know your spine and integrate fluidity.

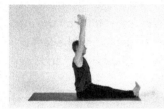 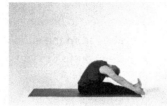 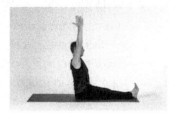

1. Begin seated, with legs extended together. Inhale and reach your arms overhead.

2. Exhale, flex your feet and hinge up and over the legs, bringing your hands to both sides of your heels. Inhale and reverse the exercise as if you're stacking your spine against a wall.

3. Inhale and reverse the exercise as if you're stacking your spine against a wall.

4. Exhale, tuck your chin to your chest and roll down one vertebra at a time, squeezing the legs together.

5. Finish exhaling and extend your arms overhead.

6. Inhale, lift your arms to the ceiling, exhale, and peel your spine off the mat one vertebra at a time. Repeat the exercise 5–10 times.

Key Points

- The roll up needs to be performed at the same speed through the entire exercise. Someone watching you perform it should not be able to perceive where the exercise begins, but rather should see a constant flow. There will be an urge (or necessity) to use momentum at certain points, but practice smoothing those "jerky" movements out. The key word is control.

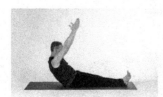 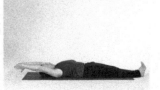

- Use the "C-Curve" in this exercise, which is the rounding of the back and spine like a wheel (or the letter "C") for the smoothest, healthiest roll down and roll up. You want to fully articulate the spine from top to bottom of the movement. This also means tucking your chin to your chest on the roll up and roll down. This exercise requires a flexible, durable spine.

- Squeeze your legs together for the entire evolution of the exercise to create more stability and add some extra leg work.

- Focus on the contraction of the abdominals to prevent your feet from lifting off the mat. I call it "flying feet". If focus is taken away from the abdominal engagement, the feet will rise and disrupt the flow. Keep your belly button to your spine on the exhales, and keep the foundation in your center.

Modification

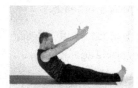

I call this the Half Roll Back. It has all the mechanics of the roll up, but you only roll down about halfway, keeping the C-Curve in the spine. Then, reverse and continue, practicing control the entire time.

Add-ons

LEVEL 1

Roll Up Twist: Clasp your hands together with your index finger and thumb pointed out and add a seated twist with your arms extended forward. Do 4 twists (2 to each side) keeping the shoulders down, the upper body tall and the chest open. Continue the exercise with spine stretch forward, etc. Repeat 5–10 times.

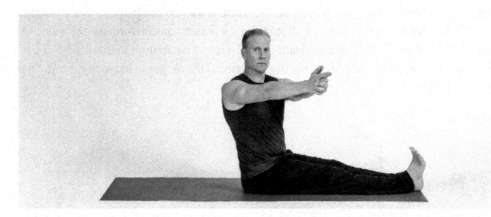

LEVEL 2

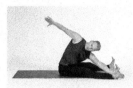

Roll Up Saw: Adding the Saw (page 78) to the roll up builds rotational power, plus adds an extra challenge to the core traveling through the movement with the legs placed wider. Perform the entire roll up exercise with your feet at the edge of the mat. When you arrive at the seated position after rolling up, twist and dive the left hand so the pinky finger slices the pinky toe for two pulses with two breaths. Inhale tall to the center and repeat on the other side, then continue with the spine stretch forward. Repeat 5–10 times.

LEVEL 3

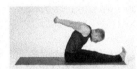

Roll Up Mudra: The mudra adds an intense shoulder and chest stretch to the roll up. As you roll up, bring your arms behind you and lace your fingers togethers into a bind. Keep hinging forward into the spine stretch, leading with the crown of your head and drawing your hands and arms behind you. Inhale, release the bind, raise your arms overhead as you return to sitting and continue the exercise. Practice 5–10 repetitions.

MASTER

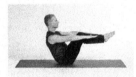

Roll Up Boat: As you roll up, skip the seated position and cruise smoothly into Boat pose with your knees bent, feet off the mat and arms to the sides. Other options include extending your legs into full Boat or extending the legs and grabbing your ankles/feet for extended Boat. Any of these options provides the opportunity for more core engagement, flexibility training and balance practice. Coming out of Boat, slide the legs forward and continue into spine stretch. Repeat 5–10 times.

THE ROLL OVER

AREAS TARGETED: Core, hamstrings, calves and spine

   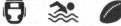

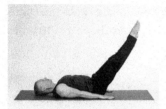 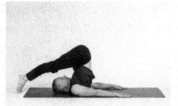 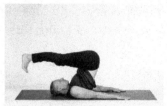

1. Lie on your back, arms against your sides, palms down and legs extended about 45 degrees off the mat. The toes should be pointed, heels together and legs zipped together in Pilates stance.

2. With an electrifying exhale, activate your deep and powerful abdominal muscles to lift your legs up and over your head while smoothly peeling your spine off the mat like a wheel. Touch your toes to the floor.

3. Inhale, lift your toes off the floor and flex your feet, sending a deep stretch down the back of the legs. Continue squeezing the legs together.

4. Exhale, contract the abdominals (belly button to spine) and slowly roll down with extreme control and return to the starting position. Repeat 4–8 times.

Key Points

- Eliminating the use of momentum is key in this exercise. The roll over needs to be fluid and under constant control, which protects the spine from any undue stress and utilizes the core muscles. The arms act as extra support and offer some assistance with the movement, but the emphasis is centered in the powerhouse (core).

- The hips stay evenly aligned and lifted through the movement with the weight of the legs not crushing your chest and stomach. Minimal weight on the head and neck is preferred. Your neck should not feel sore. I teach that the jaw and face are in a neutral, relaxed position. You'd be amazed at how much stress the face can hold and transfer downward through the body.

Modification

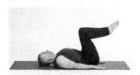

The roll over is not for everyone, so you can practice this exercise with the knees bent and rocking forward and back, keeping your low back on the mat. Inhale, rock the legs away and exhale as you draw them towards the face. Repeat 5–10 times.

Add-ons

LEVEL 1

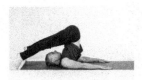

Open/Close Legs Roll Over: This variation adds an open leg posture as you roll over and then seals the legs together on the roll back. Or, you may reverse it with legs closed rolling over and open on the roll back. Keep the same strict control on the rolling of the spine. Do 4–8 times.

LEVEL 2

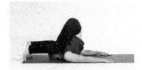

Spine Massage: At the end of the roll over, bend the knees and bring the toes to the ground so your legs are framing your face. Hold it here for 1–2 extra breaths for a deeper back and spine stretch. Roll down to original position. Repeat 4–8 times.

LEVEL 3

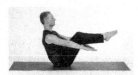

Roll Over to Boat: That pesky Boat keeps making an appearance. This variation deftly challenges your ability to control the body while flowing through a continuous movement from the roll back, up into a stable, balanced Boat pose. Exhale as you lower the upper body down first, followed by the legs, to the original roll over starting position. You are using a mixture of control and a pinch of momentum on the journey from roll over to Boat—just a pinch. Eventually you will achieve 100 percent fluidity.

MASTER

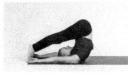

Arms Overhead Roll Over: The add-on portion here is simply placing the arms overhead, but the magnitude of the exercise will almost double. Extend your arms overhead, either on the mat or off, and perform the complete roll over. No longer do you have the strong foundation of the arms on the floor so the core becomes the motor and guide from top to bottom. This variation requires constant practice adhering to the eight Pilates principles.

ONE LEG CIRCLES

AREAS TARGETED: Core, hamstrings and hips

 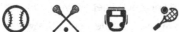

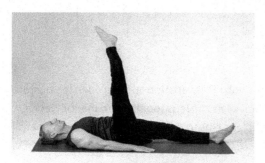 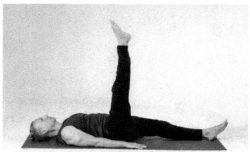

1. Begin lying on your back and arms to your sides on the floor. Extend the right leg to the ceiling and extend the left leg forward onto the ground.

2. Inhale and circle the right leg in a full circle the size of a frisbee to the right and exhale as it returns to the 12:00 position (starting position). Pause for a moment and continue doing 10 circles before reversing the direction for 10 more. Perform on both sides.

Key Points

- Sink both hips down into the mat to avoid needless jostling, which interferes with the flow. Nothing should move except for the leg which is circling. Stabilize the body against that circular movement.

- Sink the shoulders down and away from the ears. Your upper body posture remains solid while sinking the low back into the mat.

- Men may have more of a struggle with this exercise because of a tightness in their hamstrings and low back. Place your hands under your hips, and bend the circling leg or bend the bottom leg with your foot flat on the ground to lower the intensity.

Modification

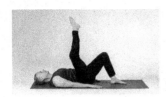

You have two options to quickly modify this exercise: Perform the circles with your knees bent, *or* bend the bottom leg and place your foot flat on the ground. You may also place your hands under your hips for more low back support. All smooth options which will keep your circles sailing onward.

Add-ons

LEVEL 1

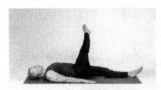

Full Circles: From the same position, increase the size of the circle in both directions to a complete circle. This means creating a wide arc which circles outward, crosses the other leg, and swings around to the starting position. This extra range of motion will increase the pull on your lower back so be cautious. You may steadily expand the size of your circles over time as your body adapts. Do 5–10 repetitions in both directions and with both legs.

LEVEL 2

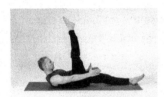

Arms Elevated One Leg Circles: From the starting position, either lift your arms off the mat, keeping them by your side, or else extend them over your head. This will eliminate arm support and force the core to work harder to compensate and stabilize your center. Do 5–10 repetitions in both directions and with both legs.

ROLLING LIKE A BALL

AREAS TARGETED: Core, spine and lungs

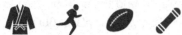

We're putting your Pilates "C-Curve" proficiency to the test.

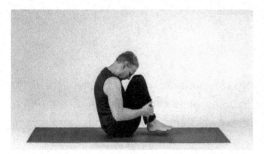 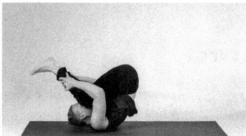

1. Begin in a seated position and draw your knees towards you, lifting your feet off the mat and placing your hands on your ankles or knees. Tuck your chin and round the upper back in a "C-Curve".

2. Inhale and roll back one vertebra at a time until you make contact with your shoulders.

3. Keeping your chin tucked and back rounded, exhale and reverse the roll back to starting position. Hold and balance that position for a breath before resuming the exercise. Do 4–6 repetitions.

Key Points

- Your goal for this exercise is to do it as slowly and effortlessly as possible.

- In addition to rolling back to the shoulders, your butt and feet need to be pointed towards the ceiling to ensure good posture. Allow your shoulders and arms to be relaxed through the movement.

- Think small. Imagine your body is a very small ball rolling up and down. This visual will help with the flow. Keep your head close to your knees and stay in a straight line up and down. No momentum, no jerky motions; smooth and fluid is healthy for the spine.

Modification

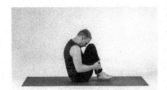

Rolling like a ball is a very tricky and unique exercise, so leaving it out of your training is fine. Rolling is not for everyone and if your spine is not rolling fluidly up and down, it's definitely not for you. Practice balancing in the original position or move into Boat pose. Hold for a solid 5–10 breaths.

Add-ons

LEVEL 1

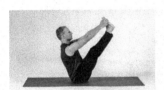

Rolling Like a Ball to Extended Boat: Continue rolling up and transition into Extended Boat pose. Hold for 1–3 breaths, return to starting position and continue. The transition requires a lot of control, balance and precision and stretches the backs of the legs while giving your core an extra blast. Do 4–6 repetitions.

■ CLASSIC BIG FIVE #1: THE ONE LEG STRETCH

AREAS TARGETED: Core, hips, low back and legs

ALL SPORTS

This marks the first of five powerful abdominal exercises, popular as a sequence and even useable as a standalone workout. The One Leg Stretch teaches precise balance and coordination through motion and moving from your center.

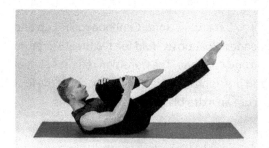 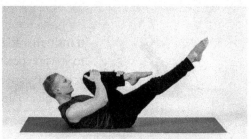

1. Rolling onto your back, place your hands on your knee and pull it to your chest. Extend the other leg away and slightly off the ground. Lift your head, neck and shoulders off the mat and contract the abdominals while exhaling. Point your toes.

2. Inhale, switch the legs and pull your left knee into your chest while exhaling, keeping a straight line without swaying left or right. Do 10–20 repetitions.

Key Points

- Being the first exercise in the "Big 5", you must focus on moving at a steady rhythm and with energy.

- Pull your knee towards your face and down into your chest with a *burst* of force. You should feel a stretch in your knee and low back.

- The closer the extended leg is to the floor, the more challenge it places on your core to anchor your low back to the floor.

- Your hands may be placed either on the knee, or else have the outside hand on the ankle and the other on the inside of the knee.

Modification

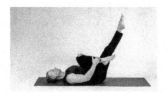

Reach the extended leg towards the ceiling to lessen the weight on the low back. You may also keep your head on the ground or place it on a pillow, rolled up towel or yoga block. This applies to all exercises performed in a supine (on your back) position.

Add-on

LEVEL 1

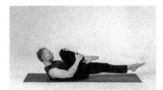

Take the Legs Lower: Lower the leg closer to the ground for more core overload. You may also add a chest lift each time the knee is brought close.

CLASSIC BIG FIVE #2: SINGLE STRAIGHT LEG STRETCH

AREAS TARGETED: Core, hamstrings and low back

ALL SPORTS

My go-to exercise for an unbeatable combo of explosive and effortless movement, core strength and flexibility training.

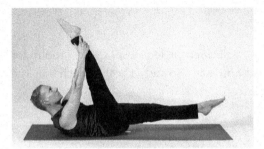 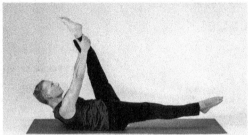

1. Lying on your back, extend your right leg to the ceiling and lengthen your left leg in front of you off the mat. Peel your head and shoulders off the mat while gently grabbing your right ankle or calf. Exhale twice as you pulse the leg towards you twice and contract the abdominals.

2. Inhale and switch (scissors) the legs and grasp the left leg for two pulses with the breath. Stabilize against the movement of the legs. Perform 5–10 repetitions.

Key Points

- This exercise moves at a brisk pace with quick changes of leg direction. Infuse that movement with breath and work on having zero strain in your core. Feel the lungs working with each exhale.
- Add an extra chest lift as you bring your leg towards you for a deeper contraction. Think of delivering your nose to the knee.
- Keep your spine flat on the mat during the duration of the movement and your elbows facing outward for more room to move.

Modification

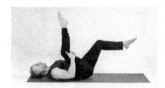

Keep the knees bent and grab lower on the legs. You may also keep your head on the mat to avoid neck strain.

Add-ons

LEVEL 1

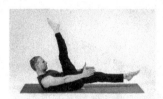

Arms to the Sides: Pull your arms to the sides the palms facing inward and perform the same leg movements. Now you are scissoring the legs and pulsing twice, all without the support of the hands. More work is designated to the core, hamstrings and hip flexors. Repeat 10–20 times.

LEVEL 2

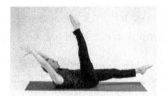

Arms Overhead: Extend your arms overhead with palms facing inward and perform the exercise. This further destabilizes the body as it struggles to adapt to the movement while you remove more methods of support. Repeat 10–20 times.

LEVEL 3

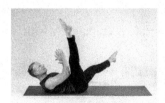

Tornado Single Straight Leg Stretch: Either with your arms to the sides, overhead, or with your hands grasping your right leg, begin this challenging variation on a classic. Inhale and circle your legs around, bringing the left leg towards your chest as you would in the original variation. Exhale as the leg is pulled close, inhale and circle back. Exhale, drawing the right leg to the starting position. Repeat 10–12 times.

■ CLASSIC BIG FIVE #3: THE DOUBLE LEG STRETCH

AREAS TARGETED: Core, glutes, hips, shoulders and back

ALL SPORTS

Extends the limbs away and back to your powerhouse.

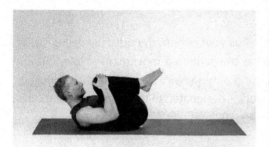 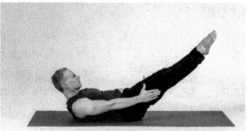

1. Draw your knees close to the body and place your right hand on your right knee and your left hand on your left knee. Lift your head, neck and shoulders off the mat, chin tucked.

2. Inhale and extend your legs with toes pointed and arms to the sides.

3. Exhale and return to the starting position with your hands pulling your knees towards you and into your chest. Repeat 5–10 times.

Key Points

- Ignite the movement from the core and stretch your arms and legs completely with a slight softness in the joints.
- Use a good amount of force when pulling the knees into the chest. It needs to be a powerful, controlled stretch—no arching of the lower back.
- Practice applying a forceful inhale and exhale, completely filling and emptying the lungs. This is a great way to pump extra oxygen into your system and clean out leftover debris in the lungs.

Modification

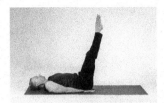

Extend the legs on an angle higher to the ceiling for less pull on the core. You may also place your hands under your hips for more low back support.

Add-ons

LEVEL 1

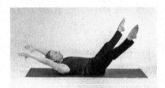

Arm Extensions: Add in arms extending behind the head to create more work for the core. Inhale as you extend them overhead and exhale as you circle them back to the starting position, pulling the knees into the chest. Extend your legs closer to the ground for more core disruption. Repeat 5–10 times.

LEVEL 2

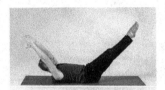

Star Extensions: This time, inhale and extend the arms and legs out into an "X" shape while reinforcing the low back imprint. Exhale and return to starting position, pulling the knees into the chest. Repeat 5–10 times.

CLASSIC BIG FIVE #4: CRISSCROSS

AREAS TARGETED: Core (especially the obliques)

ALL SPORTS

Sometimes called the bicycle, this exercise is much more intense than it looks.

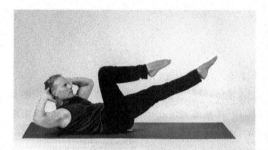 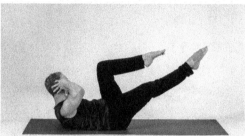

1. Lying on your back, place your fingers lightly on the back of your head so they are not touching. Your elbows should be relaxed to the sides. Draw your right knee towards you at a 90-degree angle and extend your left leg so it's slightly off the floor. With an exhale, bring your head, neck and shoulders off the mat, lifting your chest towards your right knee, creating a twist.

2. Inhale as you switch the legs and exhale as you activate the abdominals to bring the chest towards the left knee. Keep your elbows relaxed and out to the sides. Repeat 10–20 times.

Key Points

- Never, never, *never* bring your elbow to the opposite knee. I see this done all the time and it drives me crazy because it pulls the emphasis out of core and places it on reaching an elbow to a knee. This torques the neck, causing undue strain and pressure. So don't do it!

- Avoid dipping your upper body in the center while moving side to side. This disengages the core and pushes into your lower back. Keep your upper body lifted through the entire exercise.

- Keep the thigh on your bent leg pointed upward. This forces the core to work harder to lift the chest. There'll be an urge to bring the knees fully into the chest—resist it!

Modification

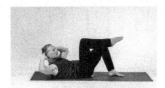

Place your feet flat on the ground with your knees bent. Place your fingers lightly on the back of your head and exhale as you lift the chest to the right knee while simultaneously bringing that knee towards the chest at a right angle. Perform 5–10 repetitions.

Add-ons

LEVEL 1

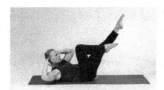

Double Pulse: Add an extra pulse to the Crisscross. Perform the exercise as is, but with two exhales as you quickly pulse the chest towards the knee twice. This deepens the abdominal contraction and increases lung strength. Do 10–20 repetitions.

LEVEL 2

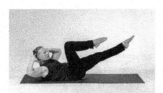

Leg Lift Crisscross: This rachets up your core's ability to anchor your body. While performing Crisscross, lift the chest towards the knee, inhale, lift the opposite leg, exhale, and return it to the original position. Repeat on the other side. Do 10–20 repetitions.

LEVEL 3

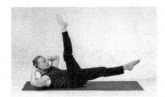

Scissors: From Crisscross, extend the bent leg towards the ceiling. Then, scissor the legs while still lifting the chest to the opposite knee. The added weight of the extended legs will disrupt the core's ability to keep your body from moving, making for a fun challenge! Do 10–20 repetitions.

CLASSIC BIG FIVE #5: DOUBLE STRAIGHT LEG STRETCH

AREAS TARGETED: Core and hamstrings

ALL SPORTS

The big finale of the classic Big 5 series!

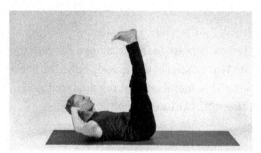 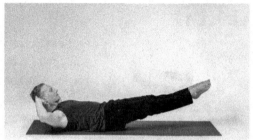

1. Beginning on your back, inhale as you extend both legs vertically. Curl your head, neck and shoulders off the mat and place your fingers gently on the back of your head with your elbows opened wide.

2. Inhale, flex your feet and lower your legs together as far as possible while anchoring your low back into the ground.

3. Exhale, point your feet and return them up to the starting position. Repeat 5–10 times.

Key Points

- This exercise is very intense on the low back, so don't hesitate to modify.
- The legs are in Pilates stance (page 23) here, so squeeze the legs together through the entire exercise.
- Begin and end with your legs at a perpendicular angle to the floor.

Modification

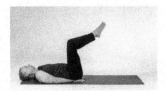

Bend both knees to decrease tension on the hamstrings and low back. You may also place your hands under your hips for more support and decease the range of motion of the exercise.

Add-ons

LEVEL 1

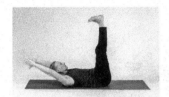

Arms Overhead: Extend your arms overhead by the ears to increase the intensity. Repeat 5–10 times.

LEVEL 2

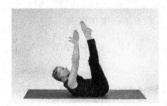

Arms Overhead with Reach: As you lower your legs, extend your arms overhead and when your legs raise up, reach your hands towards your feet on the exhale. It's still a chest lift, but now the arms are along for the ride. Do 5–10 repetitions.

LEVEL 3

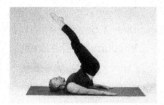

Tailbone Lift: At the top of the leg raise, squeeze deeper into your abdominals and lift your tail bone off the mat while keeping your legs extended towards the sky (it can be a very small lift). Exhale as you gently and *with control* lower your tail bone to the mat and continue lowering your legs. You may also pause for a split second before lifting your tail bone to ensure there's no momentum. Do 5–10 repetitions.

SPINE STRETCH

AREAS TARGETED: Abdominals, calves, hamstrings and back

This exercise is a wonderful example of dynamic stretching: active stretching in which the muscles and joints are moved through a full range of motion.

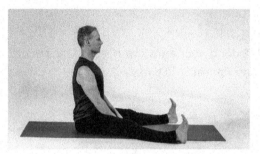 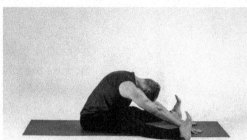

1. From a seated position, extend and open your legs so your heels are on the edges of the mat and your knees are rotated towards the sky. Draw your toes towards you and sit up tall with your shoulders back and down, chest open and chin slightly tucked. Inhale.

2. Exhale, chin to your chest, and place your fingertips on the ground. Hinge forward (into a C-curve) to the end of your range of motion.

3. Inhale and return to the starting position as if you were imprinting your spine against a wall behind you, one vertebra at a time. Repeat 5–8 times.

Key Points

- When hinging forward, imagine lifting your abdominals up and over a beach ball. This visual will reinforce moving your abs up and in towards the spine. Vacuum out the breath on the exhale. Squeeze out every drop.
- If cramping in the leg occurs, relax and wiggle your ankles and feet.
- Imagine someone pulling you forward from your hands to ensure maximum stretch and spinal articulation in the spine and back. Press the backs of your knees down to ignite the hamstrings and calves in a stretch for the ages.

Modification

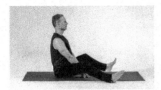

Bend the knees to release tension in your low back and hamstrings.

Add-ons

LEVEL 1

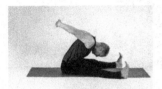

Mudra Spine Stretch: When hinging forward, circle your arms behind you into the mudra bind and lead with the crown of your head. Continue pulling your arms back and up the further forward you hinge. Release the hands to the floor in front of you, inhale and return to the original position.

LEVEL 2

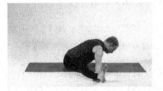

Hands Under Ankles: This requires an added supply of flexibility. Don't force the movement, use the breath. As you exhale forward, snake your hands under your ankles, tucking the chin and hinging the crown of your head forward. It's a much deeper stretch in the back. Inhale and return to the original position.

OPEN LEG ROCKER

AREAS TARGETED: Core, hamstrings, spine and back

  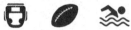

The natural, more challenging extension of Rolling like a Ball.

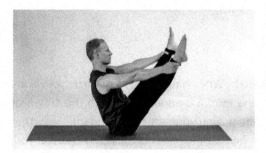 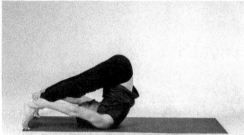

1. From a seated position, grasp your ankles and lengthen them up so they are a little wider than shoulder-width. Make a "V" shape and point your feet. Sink your shoulders down and open the chest. Find the balance of this position before moving forward.

2. Inhale as you tuck your chin to the chest and round the back into our beloved C-curve once again, and roll back to the shoulder blades. Keep your arms straight.

3. Exhale, activate the abdominals for the journey back, and roll the spine until you return to the starting position of the exercise. Find the balance for a breath and continue. Do 4–8 repetitions.

Key Points

- Without deep core strength and control, this exercise will not succeed. This exercise can be intimidating so modify as needed.

- Keep a strong grip on the ankles because if you let go halfway through . . . well, you don't want that.

- Do not roll onto the back of your head and neck! Roll onto the backs of your shoulders.

Modification

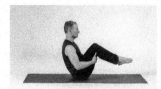

You may also grab the calves, shins or hamstrings and bring the legs wider. Open Leg Rocker is an advanced move, so there's no shame in leaving it out until you build the proper strength and control.

Add-ons

LEVEL 1

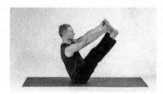

Grasping the Feet: Instead of holding the ankles, grab your feet as you perform the exercise. This supplies more weight to the rolling and forces you to control and slow down the movement.

LEVEL 2

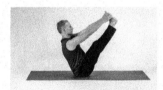

Legs Together: Grasping your ankles, feet or toes, bring your legs and feet together for the exercise. This takes tremendously more balance and control.

CORKSCREW

AREAS TARGETED: Core and legs

 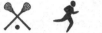

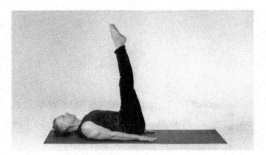 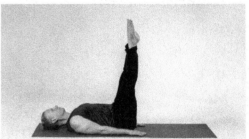

1. Lie on your back and extend your legs to the ceiling. Zip your legs into Pilates stance with heels together and feet pointed. Your head is down and arms on the ground against your sides.

2. Inhale and move your legs to the right in a full circle (the size of a frisbee).

3. Exhale as you return to the starting position (the 12 o'clock position) and pause for a second. Repeat 5–10 repetitions in both directions.

Key Points

- This exercise ripples intensely across the abdominals: rectus abdominis, transversus abdominis and the obliques. Even with a small circle, the intensity can be unbearably challenging. Corkscrew the circles with precision and control.

- Even with the big leg movement happening, the rest of your body is relaxed and aligned. Avoid the shoulders creeping into the ears and stabilize the core.

- Eliminate momentum by slowing it down, especially your toughest spots. Test this by creating larger circles.

Modification

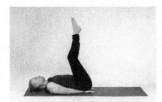

Bend your knees to release tension on the hamstrings and low back. You may also place your hands under your hips for more support.

Add-ons

LEVEL 1

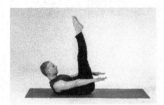

Arm Lift: Lift your arms off the ground a couple inches and perform the exercise. Note that lots of instability has now been added. You may also extend your arms overhead for more instability.

LEVEL 2

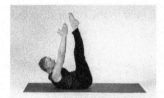

Reach to the Sky: Curl your head, neck and shoulders off the mat and reach your hands to your feet after each time you complete a circle. The lift comes from the abdominals.

LEVEL 3

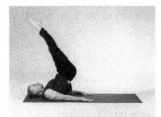

Tail Bone Lift: After the circle, continue inhaling, squeeze deep in the abdominals and lift your tail bone slightly off the ground. Exhale as you gently and with control lower yourself down. Keep your legs straight and work to transfer the motor out of your arms and place it exclusively in the core. The core moves and anchors the lift.

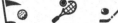THE SAW

AREAS TARGETED: Core, hamstrings and calves

This was my dear dad's favorite exercise and I always do it in honor of him.

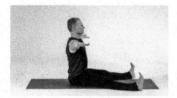 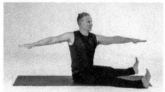 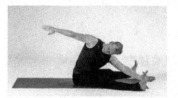

1. Sit tall with your arms side to side and open your legs so your heels are on the edges of the mat. Draw your toes towards you.

2. Inhale and twist to the right from the waist. Stay tall in your posture.

3. Exhale twice as you hinge forward and pulse your left pinky finger across your right pinky toe. Slice the toe with your finger! Do two pulses connected to the breath. Turn your head to look at your right arm. Inhale and return tall to the center and flow to the other side. Do 5 pulses on each side.

Key Points

- The Saw has the honor of twisting and stretching at the same time, which has the effect of "wringing" out your lungs.

- You have an opportunity to master the Pilates breathing technique with this exercise. The inhales help lift your upper body and the exhales assist in lengthening up and over the leg. Let the second breath on the pulse completely empty the lungs of air.

- The arms are always extended, straight and reaching in opposite directions.

Modification

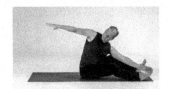

Bring the legs closer together and bend the knees.

Add-on

LEVEL 1

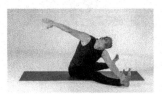

Straddle Saw: The Saw is almost a perfect exercise, so I don't like to meddle with it much. The one add-on I do teach is to open the legs wider in a straddle stretch. This only works if you are very flexible and can maintain precision and good form throughout.

SWAN DIVE

AREAS TARGETED: Spine, core, back and glutes

The workout takes an abrupt change with the Swan Dive.

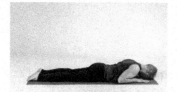 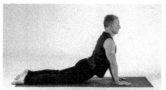 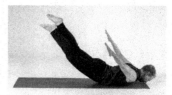

1. Turn yourself over onto your stomach and place your hands under your shoulders. Draw your shoulders back and place your forehead on the ground.

2. Inhale as you press up into an upward facing dog (see page 184) position with the chest tall and elbows hugging the ribs.

3. Exhale and explode as your arms swing back behind you and your legs lift off the ground in a rolling motion. The rolling is similar to what we've done on your spine, but this time onto the ribs and stomach.

4. Inhale and roll back to the upward facing dog position. Catch yourself for a second and continue. Repeat 4–6 times.

Key Points

- This exercise takes a tremendous amount of precision, control and flow. If any (or all) of these three aren't happening, do the modification or simply leave it out of your routine.

- When in upward facing dog, contract your glutes and the tops of your thighs to protect your low back and increase the lift of the position.

- Allow your eyes to naturally follow the movement from beginning to end. Please don't let your chin slam into the mat on the forward dive—you won't like that. Also be aware of parts of the male anatomy and adjust accordingly.

Modification

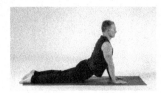

The Swan Dive is an advanced and dynamic exercise, and you might not be ready for it at the start of your Pilates journey. Practice lifting to the upward facing dog position (you may also widen the hand position) and slowly lowering back down while gently massaging the front of the body. Focus on lengthening on the negative side of the exercise (the lowering); this will build a lot of flexibility in the spine and control in the body.

Add-ons

LEVEL 1

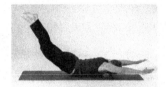

Dive and Catch: Instead of reaching your arms back on the dive, extend them in front of you in a Superman variation to add more weight to the exercise. Do 4–6 repetitions.

LEVEL 2

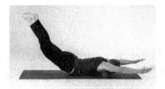

See Saw: You're going to conquer inertia with this advanced variation. From the Dive and Catch add-on, continue seesawing forward and back without placing your hands down in between. This takes a lot of core power and control to ensure the front rolling is smooth. Are you ready? Do 4–6 repetitions.

SINGLE LEG KICK

AREAS TARGETED: Core, back, hamstrings, quads, calves and arms

Improve uppper body posture while stretching the legs. There are no add-ons for this exercise, because why mess with (near) perfection?

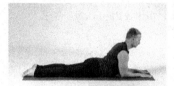 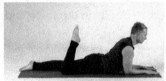 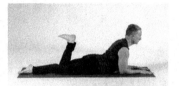

1. Place your elbows under your arms with your forearms pointed forward and hands flat. Extend your legs back with the tops of the feet on the floor.

2. Exhale twice as you kick the right leg from the knee joint twice. Point your foot on the first breath and flex on the second.

3. Deliver your foot to the mat and repeat with the left leg. Maintain a tall chest with your shoulders back and down. Repeat 4–6 times on each side.

Key Points

- Add an extra arm and forearm blast by actively pressing the forearms into the ground.
- Keep abs up and in, even before you begin the kicking. It is easy to disengage the abs in this exercise.
- Keep your eyes focused directly ahead to avoid unnecessary strain on the neck. The jaw is loose.

Modification

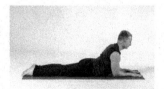

If it's too strenuous on your back and legs, hold the first position and focus on opening the chest and stretching the low back. You may also perform only one kick.

DOUBLE LEG KICK

AREAS TARGETED: Core, hamstrings, calves, shoulders, quads, back and glutes

We're adding a double kick for a burst of energy.

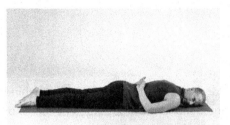 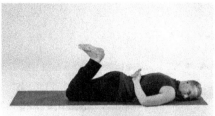

1. Lower onto your stomach, place your hands on your low back and set your right cheek on the floor. Keep your elbows wide.

2. Kick both legs twice (point/flex) with two exhales.

3. Inhale and lift your body off the mat while straightening your legs. Extend your arms behind you. Hold for an extra breath.

4. Return to the floor with your left cheek on the ground and repeat. Do 4–8 repetitions.

Key Points

- There are a lot of moving parts in this exercise, so I recommend breaking them down before attempting to rush through them.

- Be gentle with your head and neck as you continue to place each cheek on the mat. Use control to avoid undue neck stress . . . or giving yourself a black eye.

- When pumping the legs, you may touch your heels on your glutes, but work your way up to that. Allow the legs and low back to loosen up at their own pace.

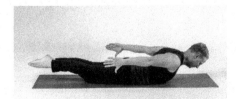 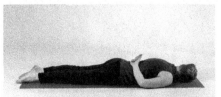

Modification

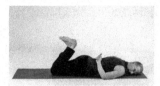

Double Leg Kick: Leave out the upper body lift and only perform the two kicks with your arms bent and placed to the sides. You can place your forehead on the mat or alternate the cheeks side-to-side as before.

Add-ons

LEVEL 1

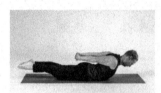

Mudra Double Kick: Instead of reaching the arms behind you, lace the fingers together and draw back for a deeper shoulder, chest, and forearm stretch. It takes more precision to grasp your hands and fingers while keeping a strong flow in the exercise. The hands will return to the low back after the mudra as in the original version.

LEVEL 2

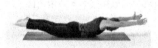

Superman Double Kick: For more on the lift, extend the arms forward to a Superman pose and then place them on the lower back. This is a much larger movement and the Superman pose creates wonderful havoc on your core's ability to anchor the flow. The hands will return to the low back after the mudra like the original version.

SCISSORS

AREAS TARGETED: Hamstrings, core and shoulders

Testing the limits of core and hamstring flexibility.

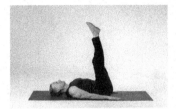 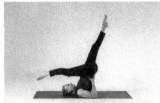 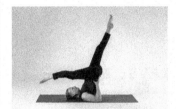

1. Flip over and lie on your back with your legs extended tall to the ceiling and arms at your sides.

2. Activate the abdominals and lift your glutes off the mat while placing your hands on your low back for support. Separate your legs into a wide and long scissors. Relax the neck and focus your gaze at the ceiling. Your facial tension must be non-existent.

3. Inhale, scissors the legs and exhale as you scissors again. Repeat 10–20 times total.

Key Points

- If you're a first timer, slow down the movement to avoid tipping and falling on your butt. The combo of the glutes and low back lifting off the floor and legs wildly scissoring back and forth can throw off your balance quickly.

- Don't move your head or neck during the exercise to avoid strain and injury.

- Those of you who practice yoga will recognize the position of the body is similar to shoulder stand pose. There's a little more of a tilt to this one as the shoulder stand is lifted straight to the ceiling.

Modification

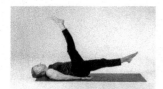

Perform this exercise lying on your back with the hands under your hips. You still receive the benefits and joy of the scissors without the heavy lifting.

Add-ons

LEVEL 1

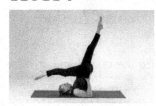

Double Pulse Scissors: Do two pulses and two matching exhales to throw a challenge to your balance. Do 10–20 repetitions.

LEVEL 2

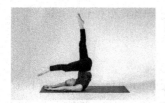

Arms Overhead: Place your arms overhead on or off the mat to remove the support of the hands on the back. This is a similar Pilates exercise to the upcoming Control Balance (page 114) but without the hands grabbing the feet. Do 10–20 repetitions.

BICYCLE

AREAS TARGETED: Core, quads and shoulders

Easy on the knees and hard on the core.

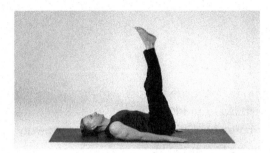 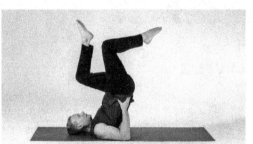

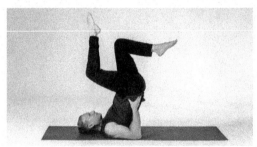

1. Begin in the same position we used for Scissors (page 85) and bicycle the legs forward for 10 revolutions and then backward for 10. The movement perfectly mimics the revolutions on a bicycle, so it's easy on the knees.

Key Points

- See Key Points from the previous exercise (Scissors, page 85).
- Keep a healthy bend in the knees and add an abdominal flex on the exhales.

Modification

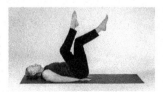

Perform this exercise lying on your back with the hands under your hips. You still receive the benefits and joy of the cycling without the heavy lifting.

Add-ons

LEVEL 1

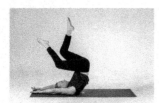

Arms Overhead: Place your arms overhead on or off the mat to remove the support of the hands on the back. Do 10–20 revolutions.

LEVEL 2

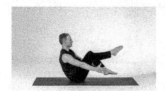

Boat Bicycle: Lift up to Boat pose and perform the cycling leg movement 10 times forward and 10 times backwards. Keep arms to the sides or, for more of a challenge, extend them to the sky. On the exhales, pull the abs up and in.

SHOULDER BRIDGE

AREAS TARGETED: Core, quads and glutes

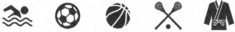

To build a sturdy bridge, we need a strong foundation.

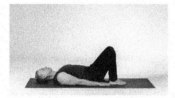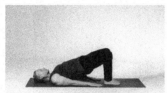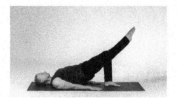

1. Lying on your back, bend your knees and place your feet below the knees. Your feet should be hip-width apart with your arms at your sides against your body.

2. Inhale, tuck your tailbone under your body and lift your spine off the mat one vertebra at a time until the weight has shifted to your shoulders.

3. Extend your right leg so it's in line with the top part of the left and the weight shifts to the left foot. Point that foot.

4. Inhale and lift your right leg to a vertical position.

5. Exhale, flex your foot and pull it back to the original position (Step 3). Repeat 10 times on each side.

Key Points

- Maintain a strong, lifted posture in the bridge through the entire exercise, and maintain a lengthened spine.

- Tuck your chin and relax your neck and face. You should feel a nice stretch down the back of the neck.

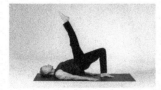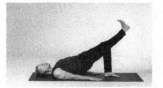

Modification

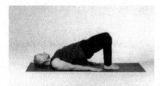

Lift and hold the bridge—with optional hands on the low back for support—while leaving out the leg lifts. Inhale and rise, exhale and stretch the back and spine. Hold for 5–10 breaths.

Add-ons

LEVEL 1

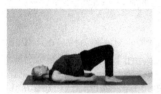

Hands Underneath: Walk your shoulders under your body and lace your fingers together. Perform the leg lifts as in the original version while arching the back to emphasize the natural curve in your spine. Do 10 leg lifts with each side.

LEVEL 2

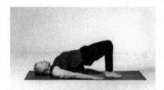

Legs and Feet Together: Squeeze your legs and feet together for an extra challenge. You'll also be making it harder to balance. Perform the leg lifts as in the original version. Do 10 leg lifts on each side.

MASTER

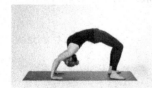

Wheel Pose: The wheel pose option really ratchets up your bridge challenge! This is gymnastics territory. Place your hands under your shoulders and lift your hips high into the air while straightening your arms. Stay lifted in your core. Now, perform the leg lifts while holding your wheel steady. Do 10 times on each side. If 10 is too much, try 5.

SPINE TWIST

AREAS TARGETED: Core and shoulders

We're really wringing out the lungs now.

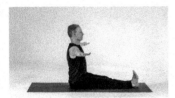 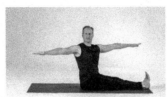 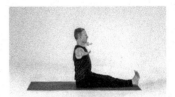

1. Sit up tall and extend your legs straight in front of you. Extend the arms out to your sides in a straight line with your shoulders back and down, chest open and lifting up in the waist. Pull your shoulders blades together in the back. Inhale to prep.

2. Exhale twice as you pulse your upper body to the right 2 times. The first pulse takes you part way into the twist and the second brings you to the farthest possible point of the twist. The second exhale also squeezes every ounce of breath from the lungs. Keep your tall posture.

3. Inhale, return to the center and continue on the other side. Do 5–10 repetitions.

Key Points

- The head and neck stay in line with the spine in this exercise and the crown of the head is lifting upward. The chest is expanded through the exercise.

- Imagine squeezing a dollar bill between the shoulder blades to reinforce a tall, proud posture.

- Minimize the movement of the legs while twisting. This is a full body exercise with all the parts working together in unison.

Modification

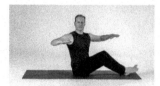

Take tension off your back and hamstrings by bending your elbows and knees.

Add-ons

LEVEL 1

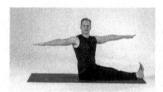

Three Pulse Twist: Add an extra pulse, for 3 in total. First pulse is partway, second is almost all the way, and third is to your rotational threshold. Practice rhythm and control. Do 5–10 repetitions.

LEVEL 2

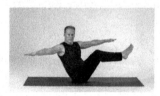

Boat Twist: Anytime we add Boat, you know you're going to have to work overtime to maintain the pose, breath and balance. From Boat, extend your arms outward, shoulders down and back and chest open. Perform two pulses in each direction while stabilizing the integrity of the Boat. You can also extend your legs forward on every twist. Coordinate the movement. Whew! Keep the rhythm slow and deliberate so your body doesn't miss a thing. Perform 5–10 repetitions.

LEVEL 3

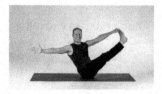

Extreme Boat Twist: This variation might just be a Sean Vigue original. From Boat, extend your legs, keeping them together, grab your toes with your left hand and twist your upper body to the right with your right arm extended. Hold for a breath. Inhale, return to center, switch the hands on your toes and twist to the left. Inhale center, exhale twist. Stay balanced. Repeat 5–10 times maintaining your balance, flow and precision.

JACKKNIFE

AREAS TARGETED: Core, spine, back and hamstrings

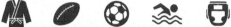

Jackknife is an advanced Pilates exercise. Proceed with caution.

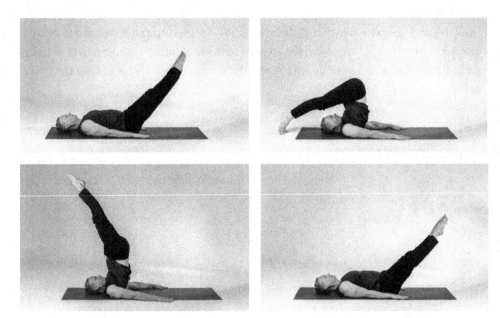

1. Lie flat on your back with your arms to your sides and chin tucked. Inhale and lift your legs about a foot off the ground.

2. Exhale, contract the abdominals and lift your legs up and over your head with your toes touching the ground as in the Rollover (page 56).

3. Inhale, press your arms into the mat, activate the hip flexors and extend your legs to the ceiling. Relax your head, neck and shoulders and keep your gaze on your toes. You are balancing on the shoulder blades. Hold for a breath or two to solidify your balance and control.

4. Exhale and slowly roll down vertebra by vertebra until your feet are about one foot off the ground. Your spine needs to articulate on the journey back to starting position. Think of it as a spine massage. Repeat 3–6 times.

Key Points

- Focus on opening and decompressing the spine during the exercise. The spine is always lengthening and expanding in Pilates.

- Work a nice balance between the core and arms for moving the body in this exercise. With practice, the core takes over and the arms are used as extra support for balance and foundation.

- Slow this one down to demonstrate the incredibly focused strength needed to maintain a precise rhythmic pace. You will have an urge to throw yourself through parts of the Jack-knife. Resist that urge, continue smoothing the flow with practice, and reap the powerful benefits.

Modification

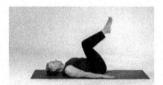

Since this is an advanced exercise, you may leave it out or bend the knees and rock the legs forward and back from a supine position.

Add-ons

LEVEL 1

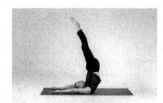

Overhead Jackknife: Extend your arms overhead on the floor and perform the exercise. Do 3–6 repetitions.

MASTER

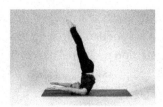

Arms off the Mat Jackknife: Oh boy . . . this variation will take all the strength, precision and balance in your arsenal, so take things slow and practice, practice, practice. Extend your arms overhead and slightly off the ground and do the Jackknife. Do 3–6 repetitions with the utmost control.

SIDE KICKS

AREAS TARGETED: Core, hips, glutes and hamstrings

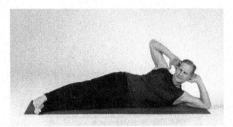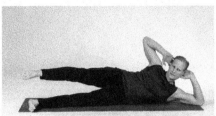

1. Roll onto your right side while maintaining your balance. Bring your legs slightly in front of your upper body for balance (you can increase the difficulty by placing your upper and lower body in a straight line) and stack them. Either place the right forearm on the mat with your hand on the back of your head and your left hand on the floor in front of you, or else bring both hands to the back of the head. Keep your head in line with your spine.

2. Lift the top leg (left) slightly, keeping it straight and plugged into your powerhouse.

3. Inhale, point your foot and kick the leg forward to the edge of your range.

4. Exhale, flex your foot and pull the leg back behind you to the edge of your range. Repeat 5–10 times and perform on the other side of your body.

Key Points

- Kick your legs forward and back in a straight line to activate the quads, hamstrings and glutes, and protect the knees. The leg kicks should be quick and controlled.
- Minimize the movement of your pelvis, spine and core as the leg travels back and forth.
- Maintain an open chest throughout the movement.

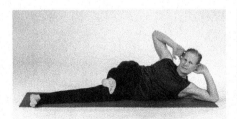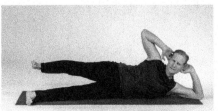

Modification

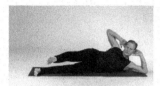

Minimize the distance of the kicks until you are better able to control the full movement and stabilize the core.

Add-ons

LEVEL 1

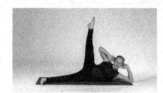

Up Kicks: Inhale, point your foot and kick your leg upward to the sky. Exhale, flex your foot and pull it down to the starting position. Repeat 10 times on each side.

LEVEL 2

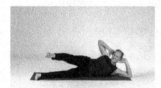

Circles: These are very deceptive, so proceed with caution . . . and copious amounts of breath. Extend your top leg a few inches off the bottom leg and circle it forward 10 times. Inhale on the circle and exhale at 12 o'clock. You may pause at 12 o'clock or circle continuously. The circle should be the size of a frisbee. Pause for a breath and circle backwards 10 times.

TEASER

AREAS TARGETED: Core

  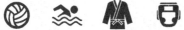

Tease your core and boost your ability to produce quick force with the Teaser.

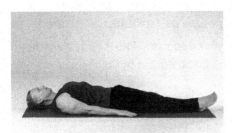 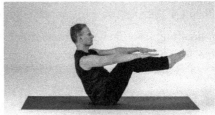

1. Lie on your back with your arms to your sides and your low back imprinted into the ground.

2. Exhale, activate the abs and peel off the mat, lifting into Boat pose.

3. Continue exhaling and extend your legs into full Boat. Hold for a beat.

4. Inhale, prep and exhale as you lower down with extreme control, imprinting each vertebra gently into the mat. Return to the original position. Repeat 4–6 times.

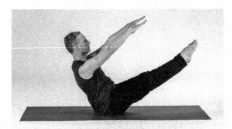 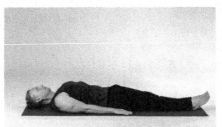

Key Points

- Teaser is a very challenging core exercise and you'll be tempted to add momentum on the lift up to Boat. Practice smoothing out the up and down of the movement and placing the driving force in the core. The spine needs to roll like a wheel (C-Curve) to eliminate any undue impact.

- The higher you lift your arms and further you extend your legs in Boat, the more the difficult of the exercise with increase—progressive destabilization at its finest.

- When lifting, coordinate the movement so your upper and lower body move at the same time. When lowering, let your upper body go first followed by your legs.

Modification

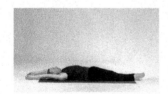

Roll up to extreme Boat instead.

Add-ons

LEVEL 1

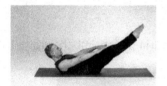

Arms Overhead: Begin with your arms overhead and lift into Teaser. Repeat 4–6 times.

LEVEL 2

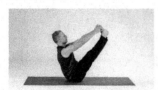

Extended Boat Teaser: After lifting into Boat, extend your legs and grab your ankles or feet. This is Extended Boat pose. Hold for a breath or two, release back to Boat and roll down to the starting position. Repeat 4–6 times.

HIP TWIST WITH STRETCHED ARMS

AREAS TARGETED: Core and hips

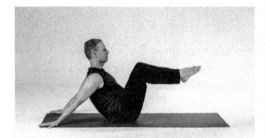 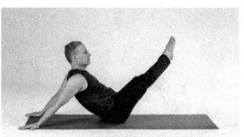

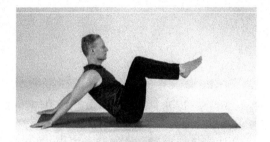

1. Sit up tall and draw your legs into a right angle with your hands extended far behind you, palms down. Relax the shoulders, open the chest and point your feet.

2. Inhale, extend your legs and circle them to the left, bringing them all the way around.

3. Exhale and flex the abdominals as you return to the original position. Pause for a moment and continue. Do 3–6 circles in each direction.

Key Points

- Practice drawing your knees closer to your head with each circle.
- Your upper body needs to be stagnant with the chest open and shoulders back and down while the legs are in motion.
- Stay deeply engaged to your core muscles to avoid arching the back and spine. Zip the legs up into Pilates stance.

Modification

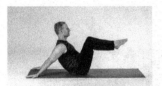

Practice holding the starting position for 5–10 breaths. This will help develop the core strength, posture and balance needed to effectively do the exercise.

Add-ons

LEVEL 2

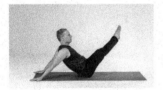

Full Circles: Begin the exercise with the legs extended and perform the circles. The weight generated by straight legs will sufficiently overload and strain your core. Inhale as you draw the circle and exhale returning to the original position. Perform 3–6 repetitions in each direction.

LEVEL 3

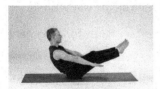

Hands Off: Start the exercise in our beloved Boat position and circle with either bent or straight legs. This option challenges our ability to balance through the movement.

SWIMMING

AREAS TARGETED: Core, spine, shoulders, glutes and back

Dry endurance swimming at its finest.

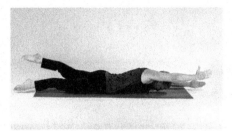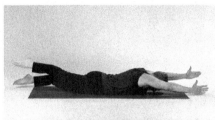

1. Lie down on your stomach with your arms extended long in front, palms facing each other, and legs stretching back. Place your arms shoulder-width and legs hip-width apart. Place your forehead on the mat and point your feet. Lift your hands and feet off the mat.

2. Inhale and lift your right arm and left leg.

3. Exhale and lower them down but not so far as to touch the mat.

4. Inhale and lift your left arm and right leg. Continue alternating the arms and legs for 10–12 repetitions.

Key Points

- Keep your pubic bone pressed into the mat during the exercise and let your eyes focus about one foot in front of the mat.
- Avoid any sort of compression in the spine by continually lengthening into the movement. This includes your low back. Reach your fingers and toes in opposite directions. Allow the crown of your head to stretch forward and lengthen the back of your neck.
- Find the rhythm between the breath and the rising/lowering of your arms and legs.

Modification

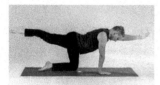

A wonderful exercise to ease you into Swimming is the Birddog. From hands and knees position, inhale and extend your right arm and left leg. Exhale as you return them to the mat. Repeat on the other side 10–20 times.

Add-ons

LEVEL 1

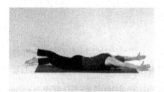

High Speed Swimming: Speed up the movement by chopping your arms and legs and breathing in a 5 count in, 5 count out rhythm. This is the same breath/movement pattern as the Pilates 100 (page 51). Align the breath and movement and perform for 50–100 counts.

LEG PULL FRONT

AREAS TARGETED: Core, glutes, shoulders and arms

Give your bum a kicking while stabilizing the rest of your body.

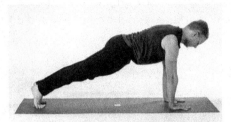 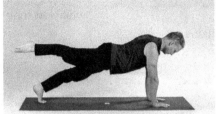

1. Assume a plank position with your hands under your shoulders, shoulders drawn back and chin tucked. Press your heels back for a leg stretch and pull your navel into your spine.

2. Inhale as you lift your right leg.

3. Exhale as you lower the right leg down. Repeat 10–20 times alternating the legs.

Key Points

- Do not allow your pelvis or stomach to dip during the exercise.
- Your legs need to be the only part of your body which moves. Avoid lifting your pelvis, glutes and low back up and down with your legs.
- Maintain a long, decompressed spine and back during the exercise.

Modification

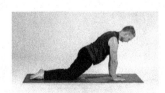

Leave out the leg lifts and either hold the plank or practice a modified plank variation with your knees on the ground slightly behind your hips. Hold your body parallel to the floor.

Add-ons

LEVEL 1

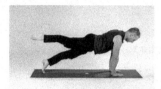

Forward and Back Press: This variation adds an extra shoulder burn. Inhale, lift your right leg and press forward using the left foot, bringing your shoulders in front of your hands. Continue inhaling as you pull back to the original position and exhale while lowering your leg. Repeat on the other side and do 10–20 repetitions.

LEVEL 2

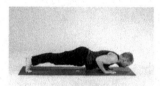

Push-Up Pulls: After completing two alternating leg lifts, perform 1–3 triceps push-ups. Hug your elbows into your sides and maintain a lengthened body parallel to the ground. Practice to failure.

MASTER

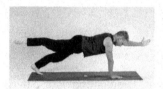

Tabletop Pull Backs: Alternate raising and lowering your opposite arm and leg. Sound fun? I have something even more fun for you! Include a push-up (or three) after every two arm/leg raises. You have no limits! Perform 10–20 repetitions.

LEG PULL

AREAS TARGETED: Core, glutes, shoulders, triceps and hips

It's called a pull, but we're really kicking it!

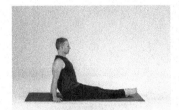 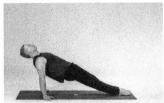 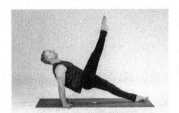

1. Sit upright and tall with your legs extended out in front of you. Bring your heels together and point your feet while zipping up your legs in Pilates stance. Place your hands under your shoulders with the hands positioned in your favored position (I prefer to point the fingers outward but I used to be a fingers pointed towards my butt kind of guy).

2. Press into your hands and lift your hips until your body is in a long diagonal line from your shoulders to the heels. Draw your shoulders back and down and expand the chest. Activate your glutes.

3. Inhale as you kick the right leg up, keeping your body stable and not letting your glutes drop.

4. Exhale, lower the right leg with control, and inhale while kicking the left leg as high as possible. Repeat 6–10 times in total.

Key Points

- The goal with the legs is to kick and raise them higher and higher each repetition while pressing your hands into the ground.
- Your hips and pelvis remain square during the exercise and continue to lengthen the spine and back.
- Beware of collapsing into your chest and shoulders. Focus on opening them to the ceiling to maintain strong posture and open breath.

Modification

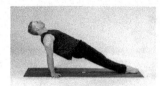

Hold the starting reverse plank position (Step 2) while actively squeezing the legs together, opening the chest and lifting the core. Hold for 3–6 breaths at a time.

Add-on

LEVEL 1

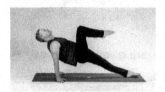

Leg Pull Mountain Climbers: From reverse plank position, exhale and pull your right knee into your chest. Inhale and deliver the leg to the original position. Alternate both legs for 5–10 repetitions.

BOOMERANG

AREAS TARGETED: Core, spine, legs and shoulders

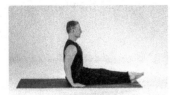 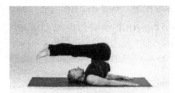 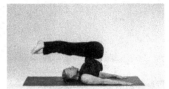

1. Sit up tall with your hands under your shoulders and cross your left leg over the right with your feet pointed.

2. Exhale, press into your hands, lift your legs as one and roll back, massaging the spine into the mat as a wheel until your legs are overhead and your arms are pressing into the mat.

3. Inhale as you switch the legs with a quick leg scissors.

4. Exhale as you roll up into a full Boat position with the legs crossed.

5. Inhale as you reach your arms behind you and begin to lower your legs to the ground.

6. Exhale while reaching your arms forward and diving up and over the legs. Repeat 4–6 times.

Key Points

- Use your hands to assist with the rollover and roll up with help from the core. Practice smoothing out the rolling motions (C-Curve) making it effortless and without momentum.

- Hit the open and close scissors quickly for an extra jolt to the inner thighs. The legs are lengthened and lifted off the upper body, while the hips are activated.

- This is a full, complex exercise comprising of many moving parts. Break it down; study it. Practice it in segments and then put them all together.

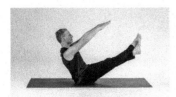 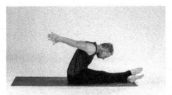 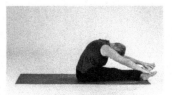

Modification

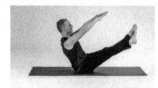

Reducing the Boomerang to a modification is futile because all the parts connect together so fluidly. Two options which come to mind are to hold the cross-legged Boat pose for 4–6 breaths, or to leave the exercise out of your training entirely. Once you have mastered the Roll Up, Teaser and Rollover, the Boomerang can be your next fitness challenge.

Add-ons

LEVEL 1

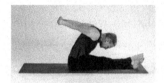

Mudra Boomerang: As you exhale and dive over the legs, reach back and lace your fingers together into mudra pose. Pull your arms up and behind you. Inhale while circling your arms around and exhale when reaching your arms up and over your legs.

LEVEL 3

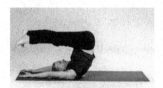

Overhead Boomerang: Extend your arms overhead on the roll back and roll up. This will remove that blessed hand support. Make sure your core is up to the challenge and the movements are supremely controlled.

THE SEAL

AREAS TARGETED: Core and spine

What a wonderful, strange and unexpected exercise.

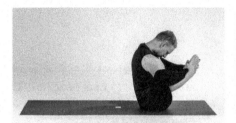 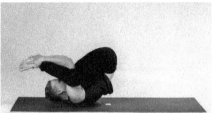

1. From a seated position, bring the bottoms of your feet together and reach your arms under and between your legs in a hug. With your hands placed on the outside of your ankles, lift your feet off the mat and tuck your chin to prepare the C-Curve in the spine. Tap your heels together twice.

2. Inhale, roll back to the backs of your shoulders while maintaining the C-Curve and tap the heels together twice again while holding the position.

3. Inhale, reverse gears and roll back up as if your spine is a wheel. Perform two heel beats again to finish the movement. Perform 4–6 repetitions.

Key Points

- Seal is a serious spine agitator. The rolling movement, lifted legs and tapping heels will challenge your ability to maintain the C-Curve.
- The biggest challenge is keeping your spine/leg relationship during the roll. Practice keeping the shape of the spine while holding your legs in a set position. There's going to be an urge to shift your legs up and down and side to side. Work on eliminating unnecessary leg movement.
- The heel taps/beats originate from your hip joint.
- Never allow the weight of the exercise to push into your neck! Practice stopping and reversing with efficiency and accuracy.

Modification

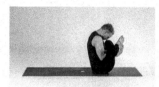

You have two options for pulling back on the full force of the Seal: one is to leave out the heel beats, and the other is to hold the original position and leave out the rolling. Your body will let you know when it's ready to move out of the modifications and into the full exercise.

Add-on

LEVEL 1

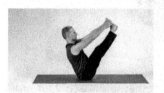

Extended Boat Seal: Roll up, do two heel beats and then lift even higher into extended Boat position with your hands on your hamstrings, ankles or feet. Hold for a breath, return to Seal starting position and continue the exercise. Do 4–6 repetitions.

THE CRAB

AREAS TARGETED: Core, spine and back

The Crab takes the Seal to a higher level of training.

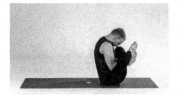 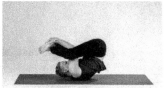 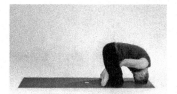

1. Stay in a seated position and cross the ankles to grab onto your feet, right hand on left foot and left hand on right foot. Tuck your chin to your chest and round your spine into the C-Curve.

2. Inhale, deepen your abdominal focus and roll back to your rear shoulders/upper back.

3. When you're securely balanced, switch the legs and grab the feet.

4. Exhale, roll up and place the crown of your head on the mat. Stay in control so momentum doesn't push you too far and cause undue stress to the head and neck. Repeat 4–6 times.

Key Points

- When rolling, continue lifting the ribs and abdominals.

- I understand that if this is your first Crab rodeo it's going to feel very unusual and awkward. Fret not; I felt the same way, but after some consistent practice I began to develop a rhythm which rolled me smoothly through.

- Beware of putting too much weight on the crown of your head. Control the roll up so it's a very light tap of the head on the mat. Maintain a strong and lengthened neck.

Modification

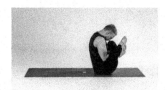

I must admit that the Crab is not for everyone . . . it's definitely an acquired taste. You may leave out the rolling and focus on the starting position. The crown of the head tap may also be eliminated if you have any neck issues or simply don't feel comfortable with that part of the exercise.

ROCKING

AREAS TARGETED: Abdominals, chest, shoulders, low back, quads and hips

We take a classic yoga pose (Bow) and add a little movement.

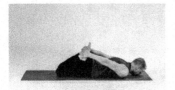 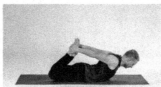 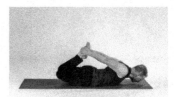

1. Roll onto your stomach, place your forehead on the mat, bend your knees and reach back to grab your feet or ankles. Your elbows should be pointing outward as you keep your knees about hip-width.

2. Lift your upper body as you press your toes towards the ceiling and sink your pubic bone into the mat. You will feel the whole front of your body open and expand. Maintain length in the spine.

3. Exhale and rock your body forward as you keep the arched shape in the spine and legs. Rock until you reach the chest area.

4. Inhale and rock back to the starting position. Repeat 5–10 times.

Key Points

- This is a wonderful exercise to open the front of the body after so many exercises with flexing and hinging. The word I like to use is "expansion". Allow your chest, abdominals, shoulders and hips to expand in this movement. Press your pubic bone into the mat.

- Your head and neck stay in line with the spine. To work opposition in this pose, press your hands and feet back with energy.

- Press your legs up as you rock forward and press your legs away while rocking back.

- Men, if this movement is uncomfortable, proceed with caution or leave out the rocking.

Modification

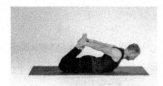

Either hold the Bow pose without rocking or bend your knees and reach your hands back into a bind/mudra. I call this pose "Shark pose" and it opens the front of the body effectively without having to grab the feet or ankles.

Add-ons

LEVEL 2

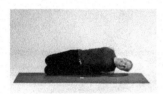

Side Bow: Want a challenge but need to avoid the rocking movement? Test drive the Side Bow—a very popular variation in my live classes. From Bow position, press your heels into your glutes and exhale while rolling onto your side. Keep the knees no wider than hip-width. Inhale, return to Bow, exhale and continue to the other side. Do 5–10 repetitions.

LEVEL 3

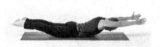

Bow Superman: This is a super strong back builder. Start in Bow position with a long spine, open chest and pulled back shoulders. Inhale and extend your arms forward and legs back into Superman pose. Don't let your hands and feet touch the ground. Return to Bow with an exhale. Repeat 5–10 times.

CONTROL BALANCE

AREAS TARGETED: Core, hips, back and hamstrings

 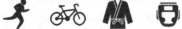

Is the most challenging of all the Pilates exercises. *You* make the call.

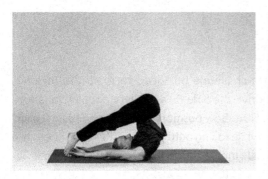 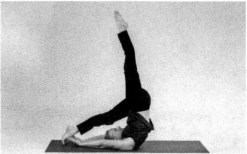

1. Roll onto your back with your legs extended to the ceiling and arms overhead on the floor.

2. Exhale, engage the abs and lift your legs up and over the body. Come to a resting place on your rear shoulders/upper back.

3. Bring your left leg to your hands so you're grasping the ankle and pulling it to the floor. The right leg is lifting to the ceiling with a healthy extension from your hip flexors. Keep your feet pointed.

4. Inhale as you switch legs and grab onto the right leg. Work on separating the legs as far away as possible with strong balance. Exhale as you switch the legs again. Continue for 5–10 repetitions.

Key Points

- As you take hold of the ankles, give them a good pull to maximize the length of the legs. Engage the hip flexors to also stretch the legs.

- Avoid compression by lifting and extending the legs away from the spine.

- Do not place the weight on the back of your head and neck, but rather on the larger, stronger upper back and shoulders. Do *not* move your head or neck during the exercise. Relax your jaw.

- Slow down the scissors and address any spots in the movement that feel rushed or uneven.

Modification

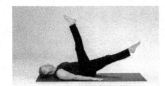

You may return to a previous modification, which is lying on your back with your arms at your sides and scissoring the legs. Perform 10–20 repetitions.

Add-ons

LEVEL 3

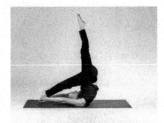

Slight Arm Lift: Lift your arms a couple inches off the mat to alleviate that extra balance. Perform the exercise 6–10 times.

PILATES PUSH-UP

AREAS TARGETED: Core, hamstrings, back, spine, shoulders, chest and triceps

ALL SPORTS

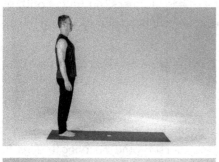 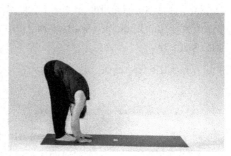

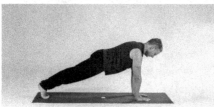 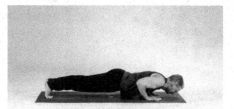

1. Stand on the back part of your mat with your arms to the sides and feet hip-width apart.

2. Inhale and stand taller while sinking your shoulders back and down.

3. Exhale, tuck your chin and dive downward into a forward fold. Lead with the crown of your head and allow your spine to decompress.

4. Continue exhaling as you walk your hands out into plank position, with your hands under your shoulders, elbows turned in and shoulders pulled back and away from your ear.

5. Inhale as you lower into a push-up, keeping your body straight and elbows hugging the sides.

6. Exhale and press back to plank. Continue exhaling and walk your hands back to forward fold while lifting your tailbone high.

7. Inhale, tuck your chin and roll up to a standing position with a rounded back.

8. Continue inhaling as you stand tall, relax your shoulders and open the chest.

9. Exhale, tuck your chin, dive forward and down and continue the exercise. Repeat 5–10 times.

Key Points

- The roll down into forward fold is a golden opportunity to lengthen and strengthen the spine while bringing some fresh, oxygen-filled blood to the brain. Focus on articulating the spine vertebra by vertebra on the roll down and roll up.

- A structured and aligned push-up is parallel to the ground. Add a little extra on your push-up by brushing the chest on the ground on the way down.

Modification

You may leave out the push-ups and hold the plank for a breath before walking the hands back. Your knees may also drop down on the walk out and back.

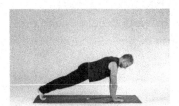 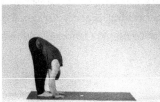 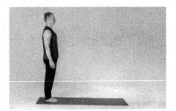

Add-ons

LEVEL 1

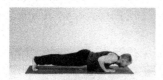

Multiple Push-Ups: Do 1–5 push-ups (or 10–20 if you want a challenge) from plank position. Stay engaged in your core and relax your elbows to your sides to engage the triceps and chest. Repeat 5–10 times.

LEVEL 2

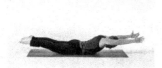

Superman Push-Ups: Get lower to the ground in your push-up and extend your arms and legs out into Superman pose. Hold for 1–3 breaths, place your hands under your shoulders and press back to plank. Continue the exercise.

LEVEL 3

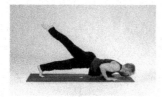

One Legged Flow: From standing position, pull your right leg back so your right foot is off the ground and all the weight is on your left leg. Complete the entire exercise with your right foot off the ground, even when rolling back up to standing from forward fold. When you return to standing position, set your foot down. When diving back down, lift your left foot off the mat. Repeat 6–10 times.

CHAPTER 5

Reformer to Mat Exercises

S o. You've made it this far—through the classic 34 Pilates exercises, along with lots and lots of progressive add-ons and modifications. But we're not anywhere close to being finished with the exercises in this book. Your training continues. I want to give you—the athlete—all you can handle and more as your body adapts and improves. We are building your arsenal of performance enhancing weapons one exercise at a time.

Speaking of weapons: you've probably noticed the Pilates reformer at your gym or club—it's a large machine that consists of a sliding carriage equipped with springs, bars and straps. Using the reformer, one can stand, sit, lie and/or kneel to do the workouts. It challenges your core, balance, strength, flexibility and control. The resistance of the pulley and spring system gives the practitioner full range of motion, added resistance and extra mobility in the muscles. It's an amazing, full body strength and stretching training apparatus . . . and it can be translated to the mat without losing any of its potency.

Joseph Pilates said that mat exercises were his personal favorite style of Contrology, and this chapter keeps that thinking alive by taking some of the most effective, powerful and life-changing Reformer exercises and translating them for your Pilates mat practice.

Afterwards, we'll focuses on Power Pilates and feature some of my personal favorite exercises for dynamic conditioning, strength and endurance training, and cultivating controlled power in your movements.

◼ TENDON STRETCH FOOTWORK

AREAS TARGETED: Core, hamstrings and calves

Our goal here is to work on getting the timing right.

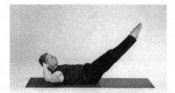 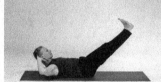 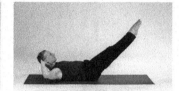

1. Lie on your back and extend your legs in Pilates stance. Place your fingers to the outside of the back of your head. Lift your head and shoulders off the ground.

2. Exhale and flex your ankles. The toes should move towards the face.

3. Inhale and point your toes away from the face. Repeat 10 times.

Key Points

- During this exercise, the low back is firmly anchored into the ground, the neck is lengthened, and the chin slightly tucked.
- Keep your hips square to the ground.

Modification

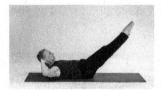

Hold the original position and leave out the feet movement.

BACKSTROKE

AREAS TARGETED: Core, hips, inner/outer thighs, arms and shoulders

   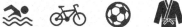

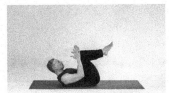 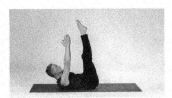 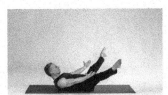

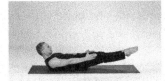 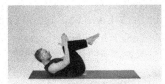

1. Lie on your back with your legs in tabletop position and your arms to your sides, bent at a right angle. Lift your head, neck and shoulders off the mat and tuck the chin.

2. Inhale and extend both the arms and the legs to the ceiling. Continue inhaling as you circle your arms and legs in tandem to the outside.

3. Exhale as you bring your heels together and squeeze your arms against the outside of your legs. Make sure to really give it a good squeeze.

4. Return to the starting position. Repeat 5–10 times.

Key Points

- On the initial upward extension of the arms and legs, reach them to their limit. It's a powerful extra challenge to your leg and low back flexibility and sets the tone for a full and complete circle.
- The lower you bring your legs and arms to the ground, the more of a core challenge you create.

Modification

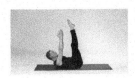 Extend your legs up and bring them back to starting position without adding the circles. Do 5–10 repetitions.

COORDINATION

AREAS TARGETED: Core, triceps and legs

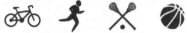

Link the mind and body to a sharp point.

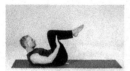 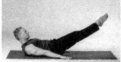 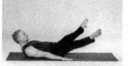 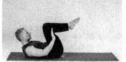

1. Lying on your back, bend your elbows at your side and bring your legs to tabletop position. Your low back is imprinted against the mat and your chin is tucked. The back of your neck needs to be lengthened.

2. Inhale, extend your arms and legs. Point your feet and bring the heels together while squeezing your thighs together.

3. Continue inhaling as you open and close your legs.

4. Exhale and return to the starting position. Repeat 5–10 times, focusing on a steady rhythm and fluid movements.

Key Points

- Hold your powerhouse strong and stable during the exercise. Allow only the arms and legs to move.

- Extend your legs to a height that you can control. The lower they are to the ground, the more challenging.

- Allow your chest, collarbone and shoulders to expand outward and guide your shoulder blades to connect to the back of the ribcage.

Modification

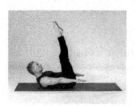

Extend your legs vertically to the ceiling for less strain on the core.

SEATED SWAY BACK

AREAS TARGETED: Core and back

ALL SPORTS

Maintain a strong seated position against the back sway.

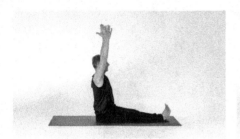 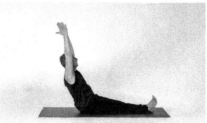

1. From a seated position, extend your legs forward and raise your arms overhead. Sink your shoulders back and down and expand the chest.

2. Inhale and hinge back, keeping your upper body tall and your shoulders back and down. Go as far as you can while still maintaining control—no rounding of the spine.

3. Exhale and slowly return to the starting position. Repeat 5–10 times.

Key Points

- Imagine your core and upper body are a block of granite as you hinge backwards. No rounding in the back or spine, and keep the neck long.

- Actively squeeze your legs together through the entire exercise to help with fluidity.

- Feel free to hold the position in Step 2 for a few breaths for an extra core and strength challenge.

Modification

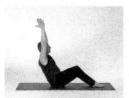 Bend your knees for less tension on the hamstrings and low back.

SEATED SIDE-TO-SIDE

AREAS TARGETED: Core, sides and back

ALL SPORTS

We add in some spinal flexion and lengthening.

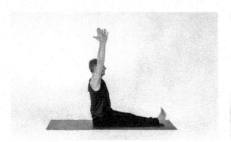 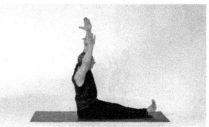

1. Stay in the same seated position with your arms overhead and your legs extended and squeezing together.

2. Exhale and side bend to the right side, keeping your upper body tall, spine long and shoulders back and down. Inhale to the center and exhale to the other side. Repeat 6–10 times on each side.

Key Points

- Imagine your core and upper body are a block of granite as you sway side to side. No rounding in the back or spine, and keep the neck long. Feel the lift from your abdominals as you grow taller with each repetition.
- Actively squeeze your legs together through the entire exercise to help with fluidity.
- Keep your glutes on the mat. If they lift off the floor, you're trying to go too far with the side bends. It's a challenge as you sway a little further to the side on each repetition.

Modification

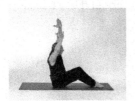 Bend your knees for less tension on the hamstrings and low back.

SEATED TWIST AND DROP

AREAS TARGETED: Core, sides and back

ALL SPORTS

Progressively overloading this series with the final entry.

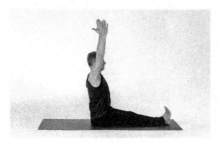 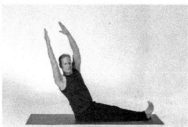

1. Begin seated for the final exercise in this seated series with your arms overhead, legs extended overhead and shoulders sinking back and down.

2. Exhale, twist at the waist and drop down in a side stretch. Maintain height in the upper body and activate the legs as they squeeze together.

3. Inhale as you return to the starting position. Repeat 5–10 times.

Key Points

- Imagine your core and upper body is a block of granite as you twist, drop and return to the starting position. No rounding in the back or spine, and keep the neck long. Feel the lift from your abdominals as you grow taller with each repetition.

- Your twist sets the tone for your range of motion so keep it tall and honest with help from your breath. The goal is to expand your range of motion more with each repetition.

- Your arms and shoulders might cramp after all these seated variations so take a couple moments to shake them out and bring some circulation back to your hands and fingers.

Modification

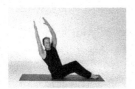

Bend your knees for less tension on the hamstrings and low back.

TREE CRUNCH: HURDLE STRETCH

AREAS TARGETED: Core, spine, hamstrings and calves

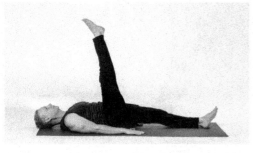 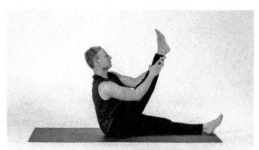

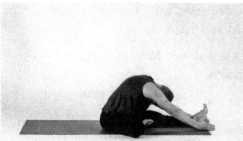 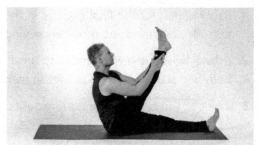

1. Begin on your back with your right leg extended to the ceiling and your left leg extended either a couple inches off the ground or placed on the ground. Your arms are at your sides.

2. Exhale, activate the deep abdominals and lift up to a tall seated position with your hands on your right ankle or calf. Sink your shoulders back and down, expand your chest and stretch your leg to its fullest length.

3. Exhale, place your right foot on the inside of your left leg and hinge up and over the left leg. Pull the belly button to the spine, draw your left foot towards you and use the weight of your upper body to "smoosh" the back of your left leg into the floor.

4. Inhale and return to the tall seated position (Step 2).

5. Exhale, activate the deep abdominals, slowly walk your hands down your legs while imprinting your spine and returning to the starting position. Repeat 6 times on each side.

Key Points

- When I teach this exercise it always has a profound and divisive effect. Some love it, some loathe it, some leave it out entirely. I believe it receives this response because it takes a lot of practice to smooth out the up and down movements. Suppress the urge to violently grab onto your leg and crawl up to the seated position. Instead, practice moving partway up and down with the abdominals as the primary mover.

- If your leg is tightening up in Step 2, practice bending and extending the leg a few times before moving on. This little bit of movement will help loosen the hamstrings, quads and low back.

- Roll up and down and stretch forward directly through your center line without drifting to either side.

Modification

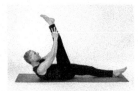

Instead of lifting into the seated position, you may exhale and walk your fingers partway up the leg and exhale as you lower to the original position.

■ TREE CRUNCH: LEG TO SIDE

AREAS TARGETED: Core, hamstrings, legs and hips

 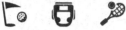

Let's take it up a notch from the Hurdle Stretch. Use the weight of your leg to disrupt the climbing and descending movement.

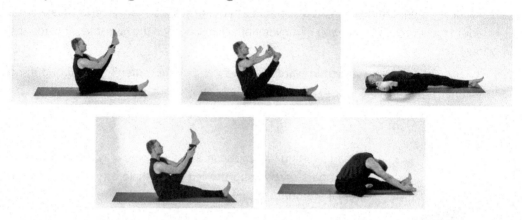

1. Begin in a seated position with your right leg extended tall and your hands on your foot or ankle. Sit tall with your shoulders relaxing back and down and your chest open. Inhale and lift taller.

2. Exhale and grab the outside of your right foot with your right hand while extending your left hand to the left side. Begin to pull your right leg to the side.

3. Continue exhaling and pulling your leg out to the side as you roll your spine down to the floor.

4. Inhale, prep and exhale while rolling your spine up into a tall seated position, once again grabbing your ankle or foot with both hands.

5. Exhale, bring your right foot to the inside of your left leg and hinge up and over the leg. Grab your left foot or ankle. Return to the original position (Step 1). Repeat 4–6 times on each side.

Key Points

- Focus on sitting tall even if you must bend the knee of the elevated leg. Your hips need to be square.
- I recommend that you master the control and movement of Hurdle Stretch before moving onto this one.
- Smooth out the roll down and roll up by activating your abdominals and using the opposite hand and arm for support.

Modification

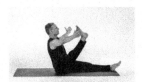 Focus on drawing your leg to the side and back without the roll down and roll up.

ELEPHANT PLANKS

AREAS TARGETED: Core, hamstrings, glutes, shoulders, chest, calves and triceps

ALL SPORTS

Expand your planks while stretching your legs.

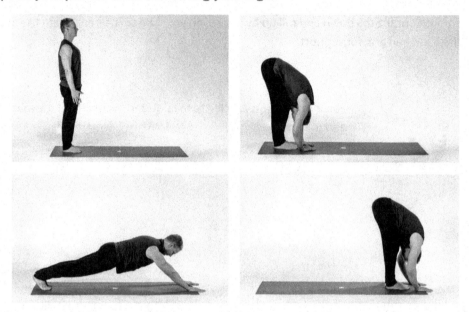

1. From a standing position, exhale and dive forward and down into forward fold. Tuck your chin and allow the crown of your head to sink towards the ground, leaving your arms hanging.

2. Exhale as you walk your hands forward as far as they will go while still maintaining the plank. Hold for a breath.

3. Exhale as you walk your feet forward keeping your legs as straight as possible and pulling the ribs up. Come to forward fold.

4. Inhale, round the spine and rise up to standing position.

5. Exhale and dive down into forward fold.

6. Inhale while walking your feet back to plank. Stretch out the plank as much as possible.

7. Exhale and walk your hands back to forward fold.

8. Inhale and round up into your standing position. Repeat 4–6 times.

Key Points

- The Elephant works best (and is most challenging) when you focus on stretching the backs of your legs throughout the entire exercise. This will push your low back to release and encourage the abdominals to support the movement.

- These are walkout planks, meaning you want to bring your hands in front of your shoulders to place more work and expansion into the abdominals.

- Press through your heels when walking for an extra burn to your calves.

Modification

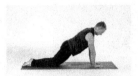

Bend your knees when walking and place your hands directly under your shoulders in the planks. Keep the pace. Elephant moves at a very rhythmic and methodical pace—much like its namesake.

DOWN DOG LEG LIFTS

AREAS TARGETED: Core, glutes, shoulders, hamstrings, back and calves

Bringing a touch of yoga with some glute emphasis.

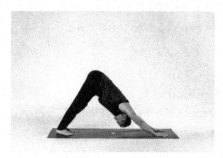 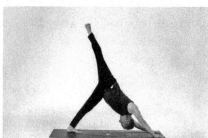

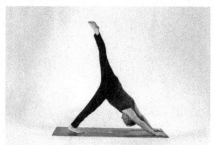

1. Come to downward facing dog with the hands shoulder-width and the feet hip-width apart. Your hands are in front of your shoulders and your feet behind the glutes. Press your upper body towards your legs and sink your heels down towards the ground.

2. Inhale and lift your right leg as high upward as you can. On the top of the lift, open your hip slightly.

3. Exhale and return to downward facing dog.

4. Inhale and lift your left leg to the sky.

5. Exhale and return to downward facing dog. Repeat 10–20 times in total.

Key Points

- I get such a kick out of bringing yoga-inspired variations to Pilates practice. The yoga poses emphasize flexibility, balance and control, and then Pilates comes along and adds an extra core, strength and endurance component. It's a fitness win-win.

- Do not jeopardize your downward dog when you add the leg lifts. If the foundation of the pose breaks down, the whole exercise collapses. Work on a strong foundation first before adding the leg raises.

- Practice moving with the same leg speed up and down without slamming your foot to the ground. I know; we really like to slam those feet down, don't we?

- Spread your fingers wide to draw weight off your wrists and pull your shoulder blades away from each other.

Modification

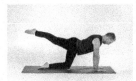

Move into hands and feet position. Inhale, extend your right leg and lift it to the ceiling. Return to hands and knees and repeat on the other side. Perform 10–20 repetitions.

BOAT TWISTS

AREAS TARGETED: Core, hips and shoulders

   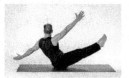

Sailing into rough waters and emerging with a powerful twist!

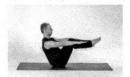 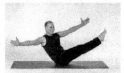 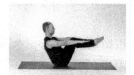

1. Move into Boat position with hands reaching forward and legs at a right angle.

2. Exhale, extend the legs and twist your upper body to the right while opening your arms.

3. Inhale back to Boat position.

4. Exhale and twist to the left. Repeat 6–10 times in total.

Key Points

- There's lots of balance in this twist, so move slowly and hold it for an extra breath. You're balancing on your glutes.

- Squeeze your legs together on the extension and pinch your shoulder blades together on the twist.

- Return to a proper Boat position with your legs at a right angle, arms to the sides and your upper body sitting tall.

Modification

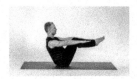

Hold the Boat position and leave out the twist, or else only twist the upper body, leaving the legs stationary.

TENDON STRETCH

AREAS TARGETED: Core, shoulders and triceps

A superior exercise for your core and shoulders.

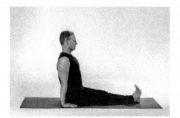 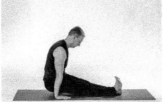 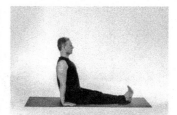

1. Begin in seated position with your legs extended forward, feet flexed and hands placed under your shoulders.

2. Inhale, press into your hands, activate your shoulders and triceps, and lift your glutes off the mat. Drop your shoulders back and down and open the chest. Hold for an extra breath.

3. Exhale and lower to the starting position. Do 4–6 repetitions.

Key Points

- As you lift, sink your shoulders back and down and expand your chest. Tuck your chin and maintain a nice stretch down the back of your neck.
- Zip up your legs in Pilates stance and flex your feet.
- For a challenging add-on, work on lifting your glutes, legs and feet off the mat while balancing on your hands.

Modification

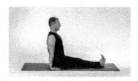 Practice building up to the lift by sitting tall in the starting pose (Step 1) and pressing your hands into the ground isometrically. Press down for a breath, rest for an inhale and press down again on the exhale.

◼ SPINE MASSAGE

AREAS TARGETED: Core, spine and back

This is the Rollover with an extra spine and back stretch.

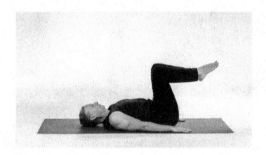 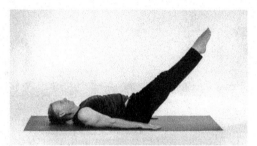

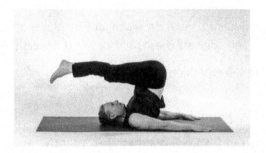 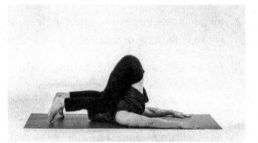

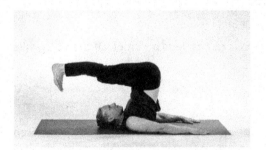 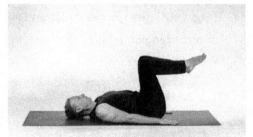

1. Begin lying on your back with your arms against your sides on the floor and your legs in tabletop position. Place your palms flat on the ground and rest your head with your chin slightly tucked.

2. Inhale and extend your legs forward on a diagonal.

3. Exhale, activate the abdominals and left your legs up and over the body.

4. Continue exhaling, bend your knees and bring your toes to the ground with your legs framing your face. Hold this position for an extra breath or two to maximize the stretch.

5. Inhale, straighten your legs and lift them off the ground. Flex your feet.

6. Exhale as you roll your spine into the starting position. Repeat 4–6 repetitions.

Key Points

- Begin the movement from your deep, strong center and avoid momentum.
- Always focus on lengthening the spine during the roll over and roll down. Focus on your C-Curve.
- The arms reach along the sides of the body and help with control and balance. Press into them if you need an extra "oomph" to successfully navigate the rolling with control.

Modification

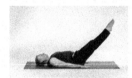

You may practice the Rollover (page 56) again or place your hands on your lower back for more support.

CHEST EXPANSION

AREAS TARGETED:Core, chest, upper back, shoulders and neck

    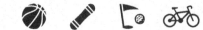

A very effective exercise for increasing breath efficiency and improving posture.

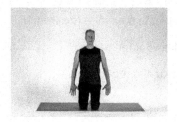 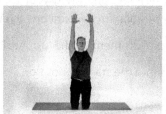 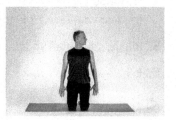

1. Bring your knees hip-width to the mat and place the tops of your feet flat on the ground behind you. Extend your arms down the sides and slightly behind your body with your palms facing back. Sink your shoulders back and down and open the chest. Tuck your chin and lengthen up through the crown of your head.

2. Inhale and lift your arms up and behind you.

3. Exhale and press your arms down and behind you and hold the pose. Turn your head right, left and forward while holding your breath. Inhale, lift your arms up and behind your head and repeat 5–10 times.

Key Points

- Keep your shoulders back and down and spine long through the movement. Pull the abdominals into the spine on the exhale.
- Stay tall from your knees to the crown of your head, even when your arms reach up and behind the body.
- Maintain a long, smooth neck on the head twists.

Modification

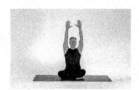 If this exercise bothers your knees, you may do it cross-legged or standing.

CAMEL PULSE

AREAS TARGETED:Core, quads, hips and glutes

 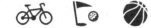

A classic yoga pose . . . with a pulse!

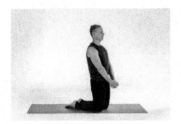 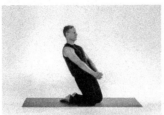 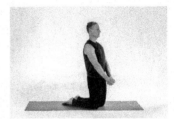

1. Take the same starting position as the Chest Expansion and clasp your hands together in front of you.

2. Draw your chin to your chest and inhale as you hinge back from the knees while staying tall in the spine.

3. Exhale, squeeze your glutes and return to the starting position. Perform 5–10 repetitions.

Key Points

- As in the Chest Expansion, keep a long, straight line from your knees to the crown of your head.

- This is great exercise for your buttocks to shine! Engage and squeeze them throughout the movement.

- The more you lean back, the more intensity you add to this exercise. You will feel a deep stretch in your quads and hips.

Modification

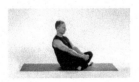

If your knees are agitated being on the ground, you may perform this exercise in a seated/cross-legged or standing position.

PULLING T-STRAPS

AREAS TARGETED:Core, back, shoulders and glutes

Turn your attention to building a long, lean strong back.

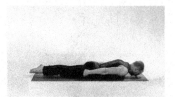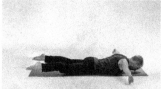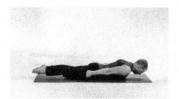

1. Lower down onto your stomach. Bring your arms against your sides and up and squeeze your legs together. Tuck your chin so the back of your neck is long and the crown of your head in extended forward.

2. Inhale, reach your arms halfway forward into a "T" shape while opening your legs as wide as possible.

3. Exhale and return to the starting position. Repeat 5–10 times.

Key Points

- Think of creating long, lean back muscles throughout this exercise.
- Perform the exercise with your hands clenched into fists.
- Lift as much of your upper body off the floor as you can on the exhale.

Modification

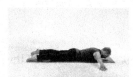

You may perform the exercise with your fingers and toes sweeping across the floor.

◼ PULLING THE STRAPS

AREAS TARGETED: Core, back, shoulders and glutes

     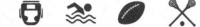

Continue building those long, lean back muscles.

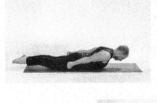 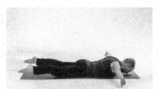 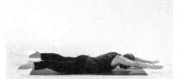

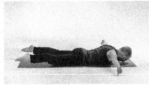 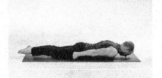

1. Begin in the same position as Pulling T-Straps.

2. Inhale and reach your arms out and all the way forward while opening your legs as much as possible.

3. Exhale and return your arms and legs to the starting position. Repeat 5–10 repetitions.

Key Points

- When pulling your arms to the sides, lift them up as high as you can.
- Squeeze the heck out of your glutes and inner thighs when bringing your legs together.
- Keep your hands in fists throughout the exercise and lift your upper body on the pull back. Add more shoulder mobility each repetition.

Modification

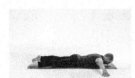

You may perform the exercise with the fingers and toes sweeping across the floor.

SNAKE

AREAS TARGETED: Core, hips and spine

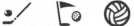

Bringing lots of spinal flexibility with this yoga-inspired Pilates move.

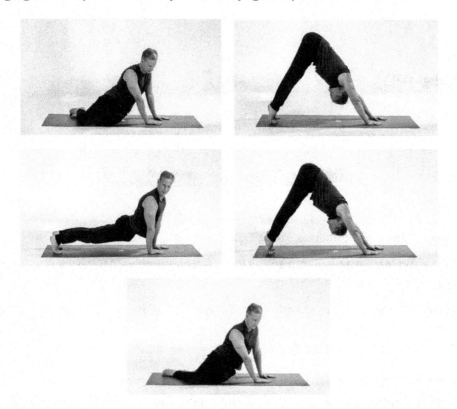

1. Sitting on your left glute, bend your knees, stack your legs and place your hands flat on the ground with your left hand slightly further forward than the right.

2. Exhale, round your back, lift onto your tippy toes and raise your hips and glutes to the ceiling. Straighten your legs.

3. Inhale and drop your hips while lifting your chest. Pull your shoulders back and down and expand your chest.

4. Exhale, tuck your chin and lift your hips and glutes towards the ceiling.

5. Inhale and lower to the starting position. Do 4–6 repetitions on each side.

Key Points

- Hollow out your abdominals and pull the navel to the spine when lifting your glutes skyward.

- Straighten your arms and legs as much as possible on the lifts.

- Squeeze your glutes and tops of the thighs on the hip drop position (Step 3) to release pressure on your low back. Lift off and land on the ground with control.

Modification

Move back and forth on your knees from Child's Pose (page 186) to Cat Stretch until you're ready for the Snake.

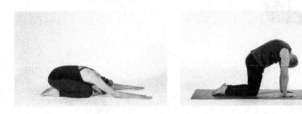

SIDE PLANK THREAD THE NEEDLE

AREAS TARGETED: Core, shoulders and sides

Threading your way into core strength and balance.

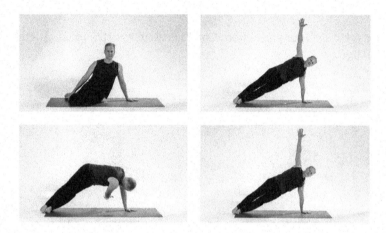

1. Begin in the same starting position as the Snake (page 142).

2. Inhale and lift up into a side plank with your left hand under your left shoulder, feet and legs stacked on top of each other and your right arm reaching vertically to the sky.

3. Exhale and reach your right arm under your body as you thread the needle.

4. Inhale and return to side plank. Repeat the thread the needle 3–6 times before returning to the starting position and switching sides.

Key Points

- When stacking the legs, keep your hips square to the front.

- The thread the needle portion needs to have a snowball effect—the arms go first, then the head, chest and ribs and finally the abdominals. Practice sequencing them in that order for a very smooth and powerful twist.

- The elbow of the supporting arm should be slightly soft and the legs squeezed tightly together. Create a long line from the crown of the head to the feet.

ROCK AND PULL

AREAS TARGETED:Core, back, shoulders, quads, hamstrings and chest

This is a severe back exercise to build power.

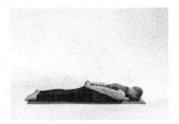 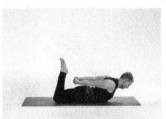 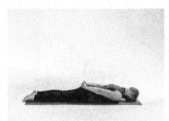

1. Begin by lying on your stomach with your fingers laced together in a mudra bind behind you. Place your forehead on the mat and extend your legs behind you.

2. Inhale and lift your body off the mat, bending your knees and drawing your arms behind you.

3. Exhale and return to the starting position. Repeat 5–10 times.

Key Points

- Work on lifting your knees off the ground in Step 2 while keeping your knees hip-width apart. Your spine will be getting a nice extension which will expand your chest and stretch your shoulders.

- Focus your eyes straight ahead in Step 2 and remain lifted in the neck.

- Allow your entire body to release and stretch each time you return to the starting position.

Modification

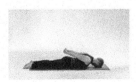

Practice just drawing your arms back and behind you without lifting your body on the inhales.

STAR

AREAS TARGETED: Core, shoulders and glutes

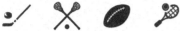

An advanced plank variation.

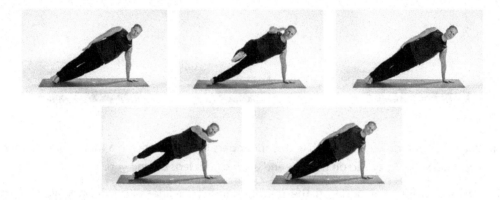

1. Begin in side plank position, place your right arm to your side and stack your legs.

2. Inhale and reach your right arm and right leg forward in tandem.

3. Exhale and return to side plank.

4. Inhale, reach your right arm forward and extend your right leg back. This one takes timing and coordination. Repeat the sequence 5–10 times on each side.

Key Points

- Keep a little softness in the standing elbow to avoid undue pressure on the joint.
- As you move your arms and legs forward and back, maintain square hips and straight legs.
- If you're moving your arms and legs so much that it's destabilizing your side plank, decrease the range of motion. Better to have good, clean form than to attempt more range of motion. "Range is for the ego; control is for the soul."

Modification

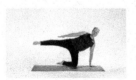

Bring the left knee to the ground for more support and balance.

ROWING SERIES #1: ROWING FROM THE HIPS

AREAS TARGETED: Core, spine, hamstrings, calves, back, arms, shoulders and chest

ALL SPORTS

Row, row, row your core . . . we're building lots of strength and flexibility in this series.

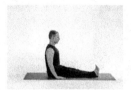 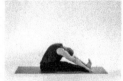 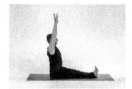 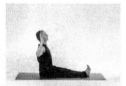

1. Begin in seated position with your legs extended forward and sitting tall. Release your arms so your fingers brush the ground. Draw your toes towards you and press the backs of your knees down.

2. Inhale prep, exhale and hinge forward while brushing your fingertips on the floor. Tuck your chin and allow the crown of your head to lead.

3. Inhale, activate the abdominals and lift your upper body tall with your arms overhead.

4. Exhale and pull your arms back and down *into what I call "cactus arms".

5. Return to the starting position with an inhale prep. Repeat 5–10 times.

Key Points

- When hinging forward, pull your belly button up and into the spine. Your glutes need to stay on the mat.
- Practice extending further forward with each repetition.
- When doing cactus arms, imagine someone gently pulling your elbows and shoulders behind you. You may hold this position for an extra breath to continue opening the chest, shoulders and breath.

ROWING SERIES #2: ROWING FROM THE STERNUM

AREAS TARGETED: Core, spine, hamstrings, calves, back, arms, shoulders and chest

ALL SPORTS

How far can you roll back without touching the ground?

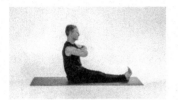 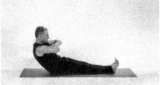 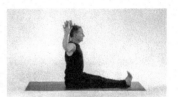

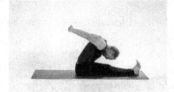 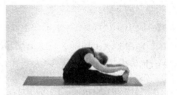

1. Begin in seated position with your legs extended forward and sitting tall. Make fists and push them together in front of your body at chest level. Point your elbows outward. Draw your toes towards you and press the back of your knees down.

2. Exhale, round your back into a C-Curve, tuck your chin and roll halfway back while squeezing your abdominals. Squeeze your legs together with great vigor.

3. Inhale and sit up tall while reaching your arms up and back.

4. Continue inhaling and lace your fingers together behind as you tuck your chin and lead with the crown of your head.

5. Exhale and extend your arms around and forward with your hands grabbing your toes, feet or ankles.

6. Inhale and return to the starting position. Repeat 4–6 times.

Key Points

- Work on sinking lower in Step 2 with every repetition.
- Flex your arms and shoulders as you roll back and up for an extra muscle toner.
- When switching the arms forward and back, expand your range of motion with progressively larger circles.

Modification

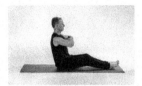 Bend your knees to draw tightness away from your hamstrings and low back.

ROWING SERIES #3: ROWING 90 DEGREES

AREAS TARGETED: Core, spine, hamstrings, calves, back, arms, shoulders and chest

ALL SPORTS

Let's get the arms involved.

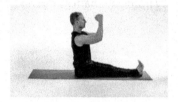 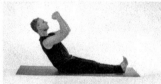 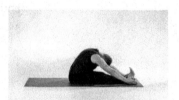

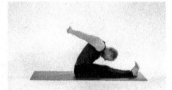 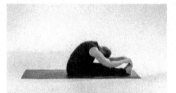

1. Begin in seated position with your legs extended forward and sitting tall. Lift your arms in front of you and bend them at a 90 degree (right angle) angle with clenched fists, palms facing towards each other. Your arms should be shoulder-width apart. Press the backs of your knees down and draw your toes towards you.

2. Exhale as you hinge back, keeping your spine long with no C-Curve. Go as far as you can without losing your upper body posture.

3. Inhale as you lift tall and extend your arms up and behind you in a circle.

4. Continue inhaling as you hinge your upper body forward and lace your fingers together behind you in a mudra position. Lead with the crown of your head and tuck your chin.

5. Exhale as you reach your arms forward and grab your toes, feet or ankles. Press the backs of your knees down.

6. Inhale and return to the starting position. Do 4–6 repetitions.

Key Points

- Imagine your core is a block of granite on the hinge back—no rounding or C-Curve of the spine allowed. For a tougher core challenge, hold the bottom of this position for an extra breath.
- Flex your arms and shoulders on the roll back for an extra muscle toner.
- When switching the arms forward, up and back, expand your range of motion with progressively larger circles.

Modification

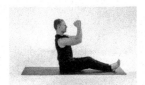 Bend your knees to draw tightness away from your hamstrings and low back.

ROWING SERIES #4: ROWING FROM THE CHEST

AREAS TARGETED: Core, spine, hamstrings, calves, back, arms, shoulders and chest

ALL SPORTS

The final rowing exercise packs a punch.

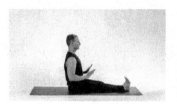
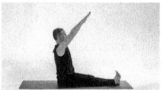
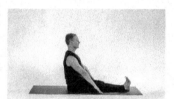

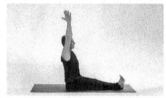
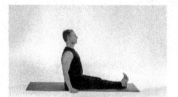

1. Begin in seated position with your legs extended forward and sitting tall with your arms bent and hands by your chest.

2. Inhale and straighten your arms forward (slightly above eye level).

3. Exhale and lower your arms to the floor so your fingertips brush the floor.

4. Inhale and lift your arms overhead.

5. Exhale and bring your arms down to your sides. Repeat 4–6 times

Key Points

- Keep your upper body tall and stabilized while the arms move.

Modification

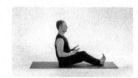

Do the exercise with bent knees and decrease the range of motion of the arms.

V-UP TEASER

AREAS TARGETED: Core, back and shoulders

     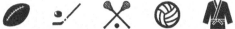

Finish this section with two challenging Teaser variations.

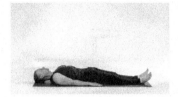 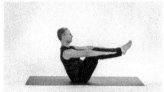 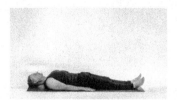

1. Lie flat on your back with your arms to your sides and legs extended out.

2. Exhale, activate your abdominals and in one strong and quick movement, lift up into Boat pose.

3. Inhale and roll back down with control to the starting position. Repeat 4–6 times.

Key Points

- Work on slowing down the up and down movements. Smooth them out, eliminating momentum.
- Hold the Boat pose for an extra breath to build balance and core strength.
- You may also do full Boat pose with legs extended and the arms overhead.

Modification

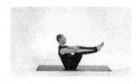

Teasers are very difficult, so do them only when your body is ready. Hold Boat pose instead, if the up and down movement is too much.

■ SUPERMAN TEASER

AREAS TARGETED: Core, back and shoulders

    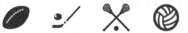

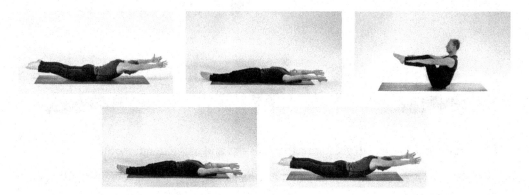

1. Begin in Superman pose on your stomach with your arms forward, shoulder-width apart, and your legs extended back, hip-width apart. Inhale and lift your arms and legs off the ground.

2. Exhale and roll onto your back.

3. Continue exhaling as you lift up to Boat pose in a quick and strong movement.

4. Inhale prep, exhale and roll down onto your back and return to Superman pose. Repeat 4–6 times.

Key Points

- Activate your core muscles on the roll from Superman to your back. Resist the urge to use your hands for help.
- You may also do full Boat pose with legs extended and the arms overhead.
- Get more out of your Superman by never touching your hands or feet on the mat at the beginning and end of the exercise.

Modification

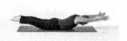 Teasers are very difficult, so do them only when your body is ready. You may hold Superman or Boat separately until you build up the strength and control to do the full exercise.

CHAPTER 6

Power Pilates Exercises

Here they are—specific exercises for extra strength, endurance and speed, all with some Power Yoga inspiration included.

These are unique, bodyweight-only variations on classic Pilates exercises, yoga poses, calisthenics and athletic core training. These powerful moves play a big role in the flows (Chapter 7), so make sure to practice them here to the point of mastery. If you can teach them to someone else, you're definitely on the right track.

Are you ready to build power in your body? Let's go!

LUNGE CRUNCHES

AREAS TARGETED: Core, quads and hips

When you train with me, you'll see I always work hard to challenge, surprise and inspire you. And here we are, adding lunges to further challenge your core stability.

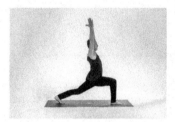 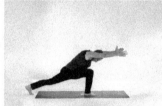 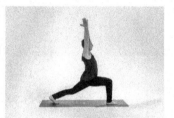

1. Begin in lunge pose with your right foot forward and directly under your right knee. Extend your left leg back with your toes tucked and placed on the floor; your hips are square and your feet are staggered. Press your left heel towards the floor and lengthen the back of the knee. Inhale and lift your arms overhead in a backbend with your shoulders back and down and your chest expanded.

2. Exhale and hinge your upper body forward until you're parallel with the floor. Pull your abdominals up and into the spine.

3. Inhale and return to the starting position. Repeat 5–10 times on each side.

Key Points

- Your legs and lower body should not be moving during the exercise. Build a strong foundation in your legs and stabilize against the movement.

- For a deeper stretch and core exercise, hinge forward until your fingertips touch the ground and focus on getting a deeper backbend on each repetition.

- Lead with the crown of your head when hinging forward and lengthen the back of your neck.

SUPERMAN BANANA

AREAS TARGETED: Core, back, glutes and shoulders

    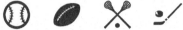

This exercise is always a sweaty, core-powered surprise.

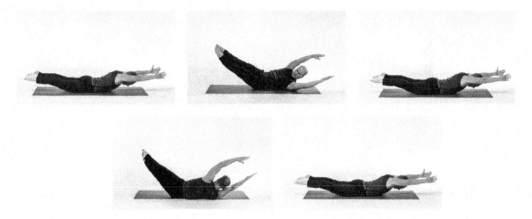

1. Begin in Superman position with your arms shoulder-width and legs hip-width apart.

2. In one big, flowing movement, inhale and activate Superman by lifting your arms and legs off the ground.

3. Continue inhaling as you roll onto your left side with your arms and legs slightly in front of you for balance.

4. Exhale and roll with control back to Superman. Repeat 6–10 times on each side.

Key Points

- Resist the urge to use your hands to push you into the banana position. Use your core muscles for movement.

- Balance on your hip bone in banana position and face your palms towards each other with your chin slightly tucked.

- When rolling into banana, let it spiral with your arms going first, followed by your head, chest and ribs, and then your core and legs.

OVAL CRUNCHES

AREAS TARGETED: Core, inner and outer legs

Drawing has never ripped your abdominals like this.

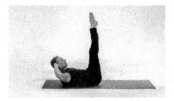 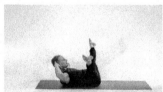 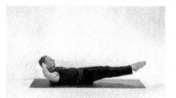

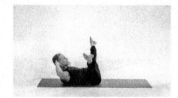 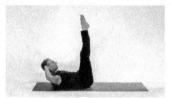

1. Lie on your back with your head and neck off the floor and extend your legs to the ceiling with your hands either on the back of your head or under your hips for more support.

2. Bring your heels together and imprint your lower back into the mat. Inhale and circle the legs out and down and tap your heels together.

3. Exhale and circle them back to the starting position. Do 6–10 repetitions.

Key Points

- Maintain lengthened legs through the full exercise with a slight bend behind the knees.
- Lift your legs up and towards you to contract the abs deeper and take pressure off your lower back.
- Add more intensity with a chest lift as your legs return to the starting position.

EXTENDED BOAT TO WRAP

AREAS TARGETED: Core, shoulders, hamstrings, calves and arms

Experience a massive core and flexibility building flow in two poses.

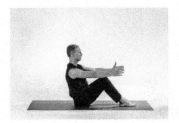 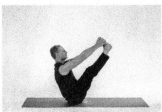 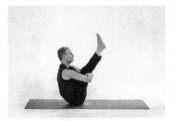

1. Begin in Boat position with your knees bent and your feet on the ground.

2. Grab your ankles or feet and extend your legs. Sink your shoulders back and down and open your chest. The chin is slightly tucked. Hold this pose for 3–6 breaths focusing on lengthening the legs and dropping the shoulders.

3. When you're ready, wrap the arms around your legs and hold the balance. Continue lengthening your legs and dropping your shoulders. With each exhale, bring your upper body and legs closer together. Hold for 3–6 breaths and repeat as you wish.

Key Points

- I see Extended Boat as the seated version of Downward Facing Dog. Treat it as such, but with an extra core and posture/alignment building component. It's a battle between the lengthening of the hamstrings and the postural readjusting of the shoulders and chest. Practice achieving balance between the upper and lower body.

- When doing the transition from the boat to the wrap, bend your knees first, release your feet/ankles and give your legs a good hug. Hug tight, but relax the shoulders and allow for the legs to continue extending.

- Wrap your arms under the backs of your knees so you have room to extend.

REGULAR STRADDLE CRUNCH

AREAS TARGETED: Core, inner and outer legs, hamstrings and calves

We're working the splits into your athletic training.

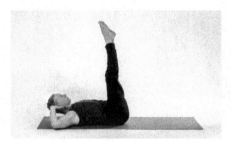 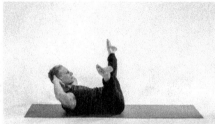

1. Lie on your back with your legs extended to the sky, head, neck and shoulders off the mat and your fingertips gently touching the back of your head. Do not lace your fingers together and let your elbows point outward. Squeeze your legs together.

2. Exhale, lift your chest up into a crunch, point your feet and open your legs as wide as possible.

3. Inhale, flex your feet and return to the starting position. Repeat 5–10 times.

Key Points

- Work on the timing of this exercise. Time it so your chest is lifted and your legs are completely opened at the same time. Also, practice the timing of the return to the starting position.

- Open your legs in a straight line outward and inward with a slight bend in your knees.

- For an extra challenge, you may also extend your arms overhead on the inhale and reach them between your legs on the exhale. Focus on lifting your tailbone off the mat.

REVERSE STRADDLE CRUNCH

AREAS TARGETED: Core, inner and outer legs, hamstrings and calves

We're working the splits into your athletic training.

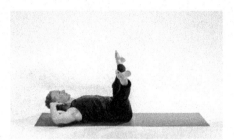 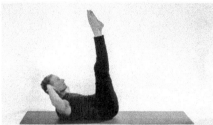

1. Lie on your back with your legs extended to the sky and open in a straddle position, head, neck and shoulders off the mat, and your fingertips gently touching the back of your head. Do not lace your fingers together and let your elbows point outward.

2. Exhale, peel your head, neck and shoulders off the mat in a chest lift, and close your legs tight.

3. Inhale, point your feet and return to the starting position. Repeat 5–10 times.

Key Points

- Just like the regular straddle variation above, practice the timing of the exercise. Aim for a full lift of the chest while squeezing your legs shut at the same time.

- Open your legs in a straight line outward and inward with a slight bend in your knees.

- For an extra challenge, you may also extend your arms overhead on the inhale and reach them to your toes on the exhale. Focus on lifting your tailbone off the mat.

WALK OUT PLANKS

AREAS TARGETED: Core, shoulders, spine, back and chest

This is a strong variation on the Pilates Push-Ups (page 116)

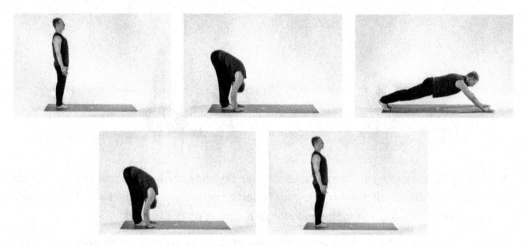

1. Begin in a standing position with the arms to your sides, feet hip width apart and the shoulders sinking back and down to open the chest.

2. Exhale, tuck your chin to your chest and dive down to forward fold, leading with the crown of your head.

3. Inhale and walk your hands out to an extended plank with your hands as far in front of your shoulders as you can while still maintaining the plank. Hold for an extra breath.

4. Inhale and walk your hands back to forward fold and rise to the original standing position. Repeat 5–10 times.

Key Points

- When in plank position, press your heels back for an extra calf and hamstring stretch. Reach your heels and fingertips away from each other.

- On the walk back, pull your hips up and the abdominals to the spine. Your tailbone needs to lift towards the sky.

SPIDERMAN PLANKS

AREAS TARGETED: Core, shoulders, chest and triceps

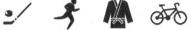

This is a fantastic core and endurance builder. Get ready to scale walls with ease!

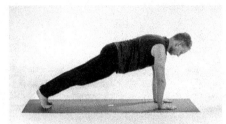 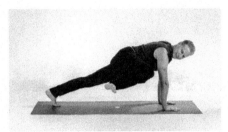

1. Begin in classic plank position with your hands under your shoulders, shoulders pulling back towards your hip bones and heels pressing behind you. Shift your plank so it's parallel to the ground and solid. Turn your elbows inward.

2. Exhale and draw your right knee to your right side. Turn your upper body and face towards your knee.

3. Inhale and return to classic plank position. Repeat 5–10 times on each side.

Key Points

- Spread your fingers wide in the plank to pull weight off your hands and wrists.

- Flex the foot of the leg which moves to your side and travel with explosive force, all while under control. The more explosive speed you can bring to this exercise, the more you will increase your heart rate and burn some calories.

- For an especially wicked add-on, perform Spiderman Push-ups: As you draw the knee to your side, sink down with your elbows hugging the ribs and your chest lightly brushing the ground. As you press up, return to plank position. Exhale down and inhale up.

PILATES PLANKS

AREAS TARGETED: Core, shoulders and arms

A plank with the Pilates moniker? This must be a power exercise!

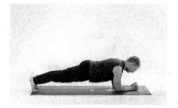 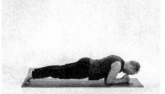 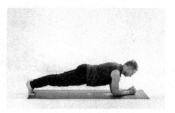

1. Move into forearm plank with your forearms on the ground, elbows under your shoulders, fingers laced together and heels pressing back behind you.

2. Inhale, press through your toes and shift forward and down, brushing your nose on your thumbs.

3. Exhale and return to the starting position. Repeat for 5–10 repetitions.

Key Points

- As you swoop forward and down for the tender nose brush, give your arms and shoulders a good flex. This is a great way to build extra strength and power.

- You might be tempted to raise your glutes up as you return to plank. Don't—instead, keep a strong plank position throughout the movement to ensure maximum core engagement.

- For a delicious intensity add-on, lift a leg as you move forward and back. Lift the right leg, move forward and down, move back and lower the leg. Alternate with each repetition.

Modification

 Shift forward and back without dipping down to the thumbs.

KICK THROUGHS

AREAS TARGETED: Core, shoulders, chest, glutes and triceps

  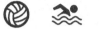

A core-inspired move to elevate the heart rate, incinerate calories and build power and strength.

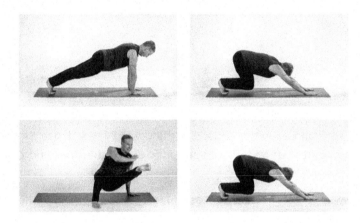

1. Begin in classic plank position with your hands under your shoulders, elbows turned inward and shoulders pulling back towards your hips. Tuck your chin so the back of your neck is smooth and lengthened.

2. Inhale, bend your knees and press back into your glutes (into what I call a "plank squat" or "frogger").

3. Exhale, press forward and step your right foot out to the side. Place your left hand on the ground and kick your left foot through, just in front of your right leg.

4. Inhale, press back to plank squat position, and repeat the kicks 5–10 times on each side.

Key Points

- The Kick Through may be done with devastating effect at various speeds. Go slow to challenge your balance, control and precision; go fast to raise your heartrate, build power and increase lung capacity; perform it at a medium pace to receive the benefits of both!

- Place the weight on your standing hand and arm when kicking. It adds a nice counter-balance and allows you more space for the kick.

- Step your right foot to the outside, perform the Kick Through and immediately jump your left foot to the other side and kick your right foot through to increase your heart rate.

PENDULUM WITH REACH

AREAS TARGETED: Core, obliques

    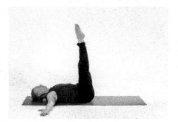

Work on keeping a steady, rhythmic pendulum movement like a metronome.

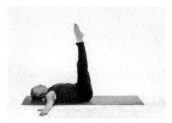 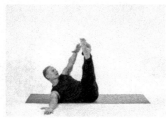

1. Lie on your back and extend your legs to the sky in Pilates stance. Squeeze your legs together and point your feet. Place your arms out to the sides and place your head on the mat.

2. Exhale and sway your legs to the right as you reach your left hand to the outside of your left foot.

3. Inhale and return to the center and continue to the other side. Do 10–20 repetition in total.

Key Points

- Sway your legs to the side, hold for a second and then reach your hand to the foot. Hold this position for an extra breath and squeeze into the sides.

- Practice swaying your legs further to the side each time. Remember to always progressively destabilize your movements and body.

- For an advanced variation, reach your hand to the outside of the outside foot. For example, if the legs sway to the right, the left hand reaches to the outside of the right foot.

Modification

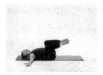

Bend your knees as you sway and leave out the reach. Keep your arms out to the sides on the floor.

REVERSE SWIMMING

AREAS TARGETED: Core, hips and shoulders

Yes, it can be done—and it's very effective.

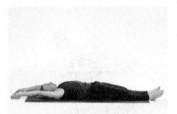 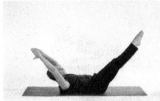 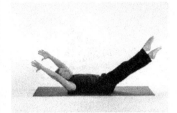

1. Lie on your back with your arms extended overhead shoulder-width apart, and the legs lengthened hip-width.

2. Inhale and lift your arms and legs about one foot off the ground while maintaining the low back imprinted into the mat.

3. Move your arms and legs in a swimming motion while breathing in for 5 counts and out for 5. Find the rhythm and then speed up to challenge your core to stay anchored. Perform the exercise for 5–10 sets of inhales and exhales.

Key Points

- Practice alternating your arms and legs slowly before adding speed to the swim. Move into starting position (Step 2) with a strong imprint of your lower back on the mat. Inhale, lift your right arm and left leg, and exhale as you return to starting position. Repeat with your left arm and right leg. Work on precision and control. Once you have a strong foundation, begin to add speed to the arm and leg chops.

- Maintain a long spine and extended legs throughout the exercise.

- The closer the arms and legs drop to the ground, the more challenging the exercise. Keep the focus on activating your strong core.

BRIDGE TO BOAT

AREAS TARGETED: Core, back, hips, quads and spine

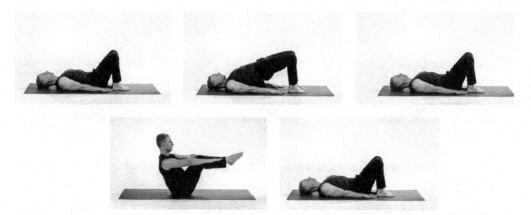

1. Begin by lying on your back, bend your knees, place your feet flat on the ground and pull your arms to your sides. Squeeze your feet and legs together. Your fingertips should be touching your heels.

2. Inhale, tilt your pelvis up and lift into Bridge position.

3. Exhale and roll down one vertebra at a time to the starting position.

4. Inhale prep, exhale and lift into Boat pose. Inhale, extend the legs and raise the arms overhead.

5. Exhale and lower down to the starting position. Repeat the full sequence 5–10 times.

Key Points

- Pay special attention to rolling up and down in this challenging sequence. Roll the spine up and down in bridge and when rising up and down into boat, one vertebra at a time. Your core muscles are the driving force and need to continually smooth out the transitions.

- Let your weight shift back into your shoulders on the bridge and out of your knees. Draw your shoulders away from your ears and relax your jaw. It can be easy to add facial tension in bridge; leave it out and save yourself a lot of facial discomfort.

- You may add on to the bridge by extending your arms to the ceiling, which eliminates that extra support. Now the pelvis and core must be responsible for the movement into bridge.

SPIDERMAN BURPEE

AREAS TARGETED: All areas

    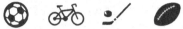

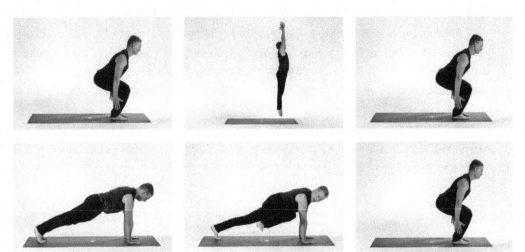

1. Begin in a squat/chair position with your weight focused in your glutes and heels. Relax your arms to your sides.

2. Inhale and explode as high as you can into a vertical jump. Extend your arms overhead.

3. Exhale as you return to Step 1.

4. Continue exhaling, place your hands on the ground and kick your legs back into classic plank position.

5. From classic plank, perform 10 Spiderman Planks (page 163) as fast as possible for maximum heart and lung conditioning.

6. Inhale and leap your feet forward to the squat/chair position. Continue to perform your beloved Burpee. Work your way up to performing this full exercise 5–10 repetitions at a time. Do several sets with only a 20–30 second break in between.

Key Points

- Burpees target the entire body and give you a great cardiovascular workout.

- There's so much to say and coach with any type of Burpee, especially this one. Burpees are perfect for HIIT (high intensity interval training) so give at least 100% to every repetition. The calorie and fat burning power of Burpees will be evident after only a couple sessions.

- Perform your Burpees like a Pilates master with a healthy dose of control, precision, breath and strength. Execute the landings and jumps with very light feet to avoid undue knee, ankle and elbow strain. The more control you have, the longer you can perform them—in the moment and for years to come. Build up all those great health and fitness dividends for your life.

- For the extreme athletes training with this book, add 5–10 Spiderman Push-ups. With this, every part of your body will be worked to overload with special attention given to your chest and shoulders.

Modification

Perform a standard Burpee. Stand tall, press back to squat/chair, step back to plank, step forward to squat/chair, and stand up. Repeat 5–10 times.

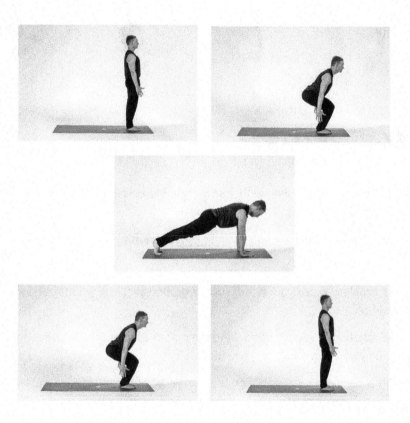

SUPERMAN BURPEE

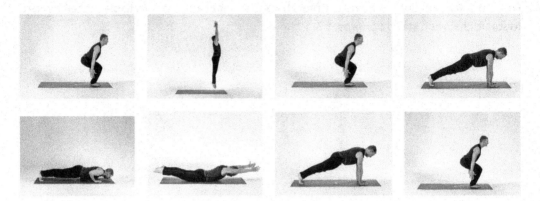

1. Begin in a squat/chair position with your weight focused in your glutes and heels. Relax your arms to your sides.

2. Inhale and explode as high as you can into a vertical jump. Extend your arms overhead.

3. Exhale as you return to Step 1.

4. Continue exhaling, place your hands on the ground and kick your legs back into classic plank position.

5. Continue exhaling as you lower down to the mat in a hover position, keeping your body parallel and your elbows hugging your ribs.

6. Inhale, lift and extend into Superman position with your arms forward and legs back.

7. Exhale down to the mat.

8. Place your hands under your shoulders and inhale up to plank position.

9. Exhale and jump your feet forward to squat/chair position. Repeat this exercise 5–10 times at 100% exertion.

Key Points

- There's so much to say and coach with any type of Burpee, especially this one. Burpees are perfect for HIIT (high intensity interval training) so give at least 100% to every repetition. The calorie and fat burning power of Burpees will be evident after only a couple sessions.
- Perform your Burpees like a Pilates master with a healthy dose of control, precision, breath and strength. Execute the landings and jumps with very light feet to avoid undue knee, ankle and elbow strain. The more control you have, the longer you can perform them—in the moment and for years to come. Build up all those great health and fitness dividends for your life.
- Extend your Superman pose completely. Lengthen so much that your fingers and toes feel 5 miles apart with your back feeling impervious.

Modification

Perform a standard Burpee. Stand tall, press back to squat/chair, step back to plank, step forward to squat/chair, and stand up. Repeat 5–10 times.

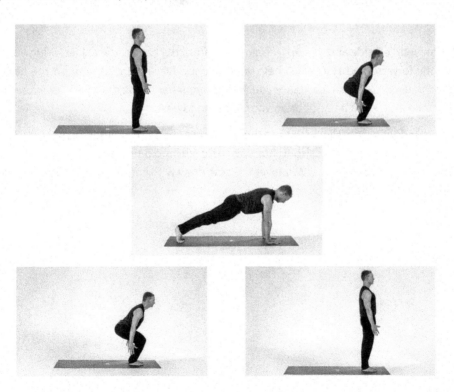

SIDE LEG SERIES #1: CIRCLES

AREAS TARGETED: Core, hips and thighs

ALL SPORTS

This series is deceptively challenging and causes many of my athletes to tap out early. My advice for a successful Side Leg Series is to stabilize your core against the movements of the legs with the hips stacked. You may also do this series from a kneeling side kick position. Place your hand and knee on the ground with the targeted leg lengthened parallel to the floor (see the images below). Perform these exercises on both sides of your body.

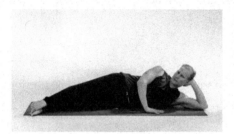 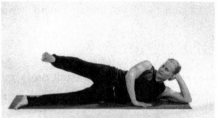

1. Lie on your left side and line up a straight line from the ears to the ankles. Bring your legs slightly forward and stacked to help with balance. Place your left arm on the floor and bend your elbow so you can place your head in your hand. The right hand is placed on the mat for a little extra balance or on your right hip for less.

2. Lift your right leg parallel with the ground. Circle it forward 10 times, drawing a circle the size of a frisbee. You may also tighten up the circle into a tiny one or hit the boundaries and go for a very wide one. Whatever the size, draw with control and precision. Circle the leg 10 times in the other direction.

SIDE LEG SERIES #2: TAPS

AREAS TARGETED: Core, hips and thighs

ALL SPORTS

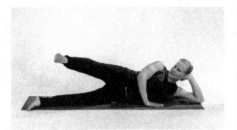 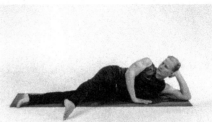

1. Lie on your left side and line up a straight line from the ears to the ankles. Bring your legs slightly forward and stacked to help with balance. Place your left arm on the floor and bend your elbow so you can place your head in your hand. The right hand is placed on the mat for a little extra balance or on your right hip for less.

2. Inhale and lift your right leg parallel with the ground. Exhale and tap your toes in front of you.

3. Inhale and swing your leg behind you and give a light tap. Swoop the leg high in the center and bring it down with beautiful control on the taps. Do 10–20 repetitions in total.

■ SIDE LEG SERIES #3: KICKS

AREAS TARGETED: Core, hips and thighs

ALL SPORTS

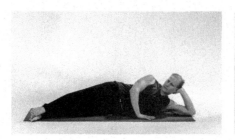 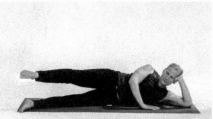

1. Lie on your left side and line up a straight line from the ears to the ankles. Bring your legs slightly forward and stacked to help with balance. Place your left arm on the floor and bend your elbow so you can place your head in your hand. The right hand is placed on the mat for a little extra balance or on your right hip for less.

2. Lift your right leg parallel with the ground. Point your right foot, inhale and kick your leg forward in a straight line.

3. Exhale, flex your foot and pull it back behind you, maintaining the straight line. Do 10–20 repetitions.

SIDE LEG SERIES #4: TRIANGLES

AREAS TARGETED: Core, hips and thighs

ALL SPORTS

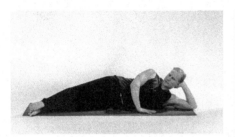 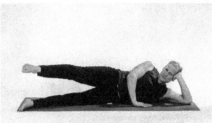

1. Lie on your left side and line up a straight line from the ears to the ankles. Bring your legs slightly forward and stacked to help with balance. Place your left arm on the floor and bend your elbow so you can place your head in your hand. The right hand is placed on the mat for a little extra balance or on your right hip for less.

2. Lift your right leg parallel to the ground. Draw a triangle in one direction 10 times. Make is as precise as possible (which in my experience is easier said than done). After about 3 repetitions, the triangle will likely resemble a blobby mess, but stay focused on sketching that triangle no matter what begins to happen with your legs, hips and core. Draw the triangle in the opposite direction 10 times.

SIDE LEG SERIES #5: THE "U" SWING

AREAS TARGETED: Core, hips and thighs

ALL SPORTS

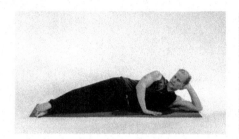 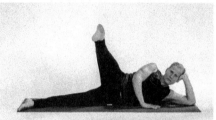

1. Lie on your left side and line up a straight line from the ears to the ankles. Bring your legs slightly forward and stacked to help with balance. Place your left arm on the floor and bend your elbow so you can place your head in your hand. The right hand is placed on the mat for a little extra balance or on your right hip for less.

2. Lift your right leg parallel to the ground. Inhale and sweep the leg forward and up.

3. Exhale and pull the leg back and up. You have now drawn the letter "U". Do 10–20 repetitions.

SIDE LEG SERIES #6: KICK UPS

AREAS TARGETED: Core, hips and thighs

ALL SPORTS

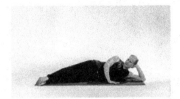 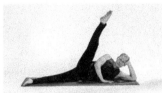 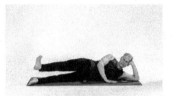

1. Lie on your left side and line up a straight line from the ears to the ankles. Bring your legs slightly forward and stacked to help with balance. Place your left arm on the floor and bend your elbow so you can place your head in your hand. The right hand is placed on the mat for a little extra balance or on your right hip for less.

2. Inhale, point your right foot and kick your right leg to the sky.

3. Exhale, flex your foot and lower your leg with control. Do 6–10 repetitions.

Key Points

- The Side Leg series (as you can now see/feel) is a killer! To someone watching you perform these exercises, it might look easy. "What's the big deal? It's just a few circles and kicks." But the amount of precision and intensity required can very quickly tax your muscles and reserves. This is why the discipline and dedication of your Pilates practice must always be 100%. To do less is a disservice to you and this wonderful training program. This series is a severe reminder about why we do Pilates: strength, flexibility, endurance, control, precision and power.

- Imagine moving your leg through something murky and thick, like peanut butter or pudding. Train your mind to add resistance to these bodyweight exercises and you can achieve a deeper muscle engagement.

- Your upper body is to remain motionless throughout every one of the six side leg variations—no movement above the waist. When your upper body is still and stabilized, you will receive extra strength and mobility benefits in your core, glutes, legs and hips.

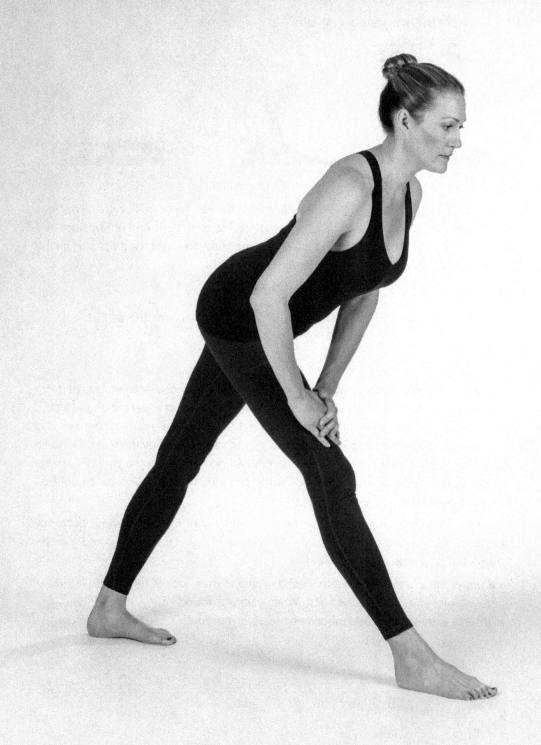

CHAPTER 7

Cool Down Stretches

Be patient; we're almost at the flows!

I've added some very effective yoga poses and stretch exercises for you to do after any of the flows found in Chapter 7. These may be done as stand-alone sequences for total body release and restoration, or even after your regular athletic conditioning—be it weight training, kettlebell exercises, sprints, scrimmages, HIIT, power lifting or running drills. They are appropriate for all athletes, and applicable for all sports.

I am also very excited to include yoga in this book, since Pilates and yoga work so brilliantly together. Pilates enhances the core and body through dynamic movements and yoga focuses on flexibility (and much more) through held poses and sequences.

Stretching regularly also has numerous benefits that increase your overall athletic performance, including:

1. Increased flexibility
2. Increased muscle mobility
3. Supplying more fresh blood and oxygen to the muscles, which increases energy levels
4. Reduced musculoskeletal pain and improved body alignment
5. Reduced back pain and discomfort
6. Reduced mental, emotional and physical stress
7. Increased range of motion in the joints
8. Reduced risk of injury

CHILD'S POSE

AREAS TARGETED: Low back, spine, glutes, shoulders, hips

Soothe your back and catch your breath. My son does this pose with ease.

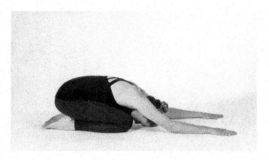

1. Place your knees hip-width apart on the floor and walk your hands forward as you sink your glutes back and down onto the heels.

2. Relax your shoulders back and release your forehead to the mat. You may also place your arms to your sides for less of a back and spine stretch. Square your hips and spread your fingers wide. Hold for 5–10 deep breaths and allow your body to completely relax.

Key Points

- Child's Pose is a wonderful pose for calming the mind and releasing the body through gentle yet profound stretching. It is easily accessible any time during your Pilates workouts when you need a moment to regroup, release and bring the focus back to your breath.

- Lengthen this pose by pressing your tailbone back and reaching your fingers forward while drawing your shoulders back and down. You may walk your hands further forward, lift your glutes slightly off your heels and sink your chest towards the floor in what is known as the Puppy Pose. This pose really enhances the natural curve in the spine and expands the shoulders.

- This is a huge favorite with my live classes and online videos. Whenever I mention it's time for Child's Pose, everyone collectively smiles, sighs and moves immediately into the pose. They don't need to be told twice, and neither will you.

Modification

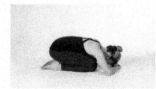

You may rest your head on your hands or fists or use a block for additional head and neck support. Place a rolled-up towel or blanket under your knees for a softer surface.

COBRA

AREAS TARGETED: Glutes, spine, back, chest, shoulders, triceps and hips

Open the flexibility in your back and spine with these backbends.

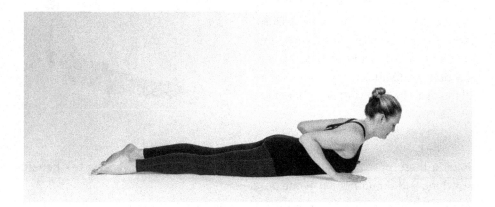

1. Lie on your stomach and place your hands under your shoulders with your elbows hugging the ribs. Extend your legs behind you with the tops of your feet on the mat.

2. Inhale and lift your upper body while drawing your shoulders back and down and expanding your chest. Focus on lengthening from the crown of your head through the tips of your toes. Squeeze your glutes and quads to offer more support to the lower back. Hold for 5–10 deep breaths.

UPWARD FACING DOG

AREAS TARGETED: Chest, shoulders, abs, wrists, arms and glutes

1. From Cobra, inhale and lift the upper body so your arms are straight (with a tiny bit of softness in the elbows). Draw your shoulders back and down and expand your chest. Squeeze your glutes and quads and lift your legs and knees off the mat. Hold for 5–10 deep breaths.

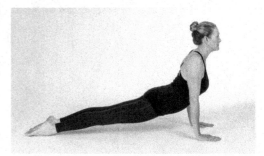

Key Points

- Holding these poses really strengthens the upper body. You receive the benefits of stretching and strengthening in one pose.

- These poses allow for much better and more open breathing, so make sure your shoulders are down and your chest is opening and expanding. It might feel very strange to open your chest like this if you're used to having shoulders which roll forward all day, but it's essential. Proper posture will encourage maximum oxygen flow.

- If you're an athlete who spends many hours in a seated or deep squat position, these poses will bring mobility to your back and hips while lifting your overall posture.

PIGEON

AREAS TARGETED: Hips, back, glutes and shoulders
One of the most beloved stretches and a mid-level popularity bird.

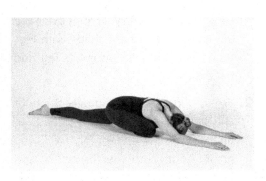

1. From Downward Facing Dog (page 43), exhale and bring your right knee forward and onto the ground. Place your hands under your shoulders and lift tall as you square your hips, slide your left leg back and open your right leg. Place your weight right over the center of the pose and walk your hands forward. Release your upper body and soak up this beautiful stretch. Hold for 10–15 breaths on each side.

Key Points

- Your hips store up so much tension, tightness and stress that it affects the rest of your body. Pigeon pose is legendary for unlocking the hips and the surrounding area. Practicing it every day will bring more mobility and release.

- As you add more Pigeon to your training, walk your front foot forward as your body allows. The goal is to bring your front leg into a right angle for optimum knee, hip, glute and back release.

- Practice holding Proud Pigeon first, with hands on the mat and lifting the upper body while sinking your shoulders back and down and expanding your chest. Feel the added stretch in your abdominals and chest. You will also receive a nice contraction in your shoulders and triceps.

Modification

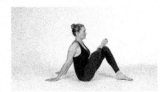

Not ready for Pigeon? Do Seated Pigeon: Sit down, extend your left leg, bend your right leg and place your right ankle on the left thigh. Bend your left knee and place your left foot on the mat. Bring your hands to the mat behind you and press forward while exhaling. Repeat on both sides.

SCORPION

AREAS TARGETED: Hips, abdominals, back and quads
This is a favorite for back flexibility.

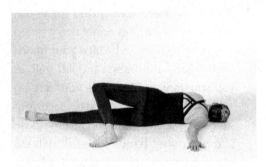

1. Lie on your back with your arms extended out to the sides in a T-shape with legs together. Inhale, lift your left leg and bend the knee.

2. Exhale and cross that leg over the right and slide your foot onto the floor. Continue to slide the left foot forward as you breathe out. Keep your hands flat and focus on twisting from your low back. Repeat on both sides for 10–15 breaths.

Key Points

- Scorpion is an upside down Lying Spinal Twist (page 192) and can work wonders for releasing tight and stubborn back muscles so your circulation will flow again.

- This stretch is very effective at connecting with your sore glutes and tight hip flexors. Too much sitting, crouching and standing weakens your glute/hip flexor connection and the Scorpion is the key to untying them.

- You may also extend your arms overhead for more length in the twist.

PYRAMID

AREAS TARGETED: Hamstrings, spine, hips, back and calves, balance and alignment

The Pyramid combines deep focus with a surprising balance challenge.

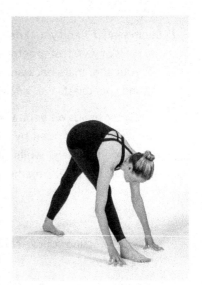

1. From a standing position, step your right foot forward about 3–4 feet and place your hands on your hips. Your feet are not in a straight line but are slightly staggered. Make sure your hips are square and your shoulders back and down. The chest is open and expanded.

2. Tuck your chin slightly and lengthen the back of your neck. Exhale and hinge your upper body up and over your right leg until you can place your hands on the mat to the sides of your right foot.

3. With each exhale, lengthen your legs and hinge forward from your chest to your navel. Draw your nose towards your right knee. Continue holding this pose for 5–10 breaths and repeat on the other side.

Key Points

- Continuously exten;/,d from the crown of your head while your tailbone reaches back behind you.

- Make sure both your feet are always pointed forwards. The back foot can have a tendency to wander into an open turnout position. Press both heels down with each exhale to maintain strong feet position.

- For an add-on, reach your arms behind and lace your fingers together into a mudra pose with your palms squeezing together. Continue hinging forward while simultaneously drawing your hands, arms, shoulders and chest back.

Modification

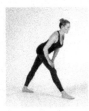

Instead of bringing your hands all the way to the floor, place them on your leg for more support and less intensity on your back and legs. You can place them on your quad and slowly walk your fingers down with each exhale.

■ BUTTERFLY

AREAS TARGETED: Inner thighs, hips, groin, hamstrings and knees

ALL SPORTS

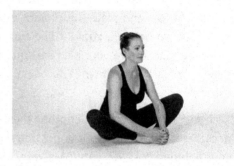

1. Begin seated, bend your knees and bring the soles of your feet together. Sit up tall, roll your shoulders back and down and expand your chest.

2. Place your hands on your ankles or feet and pry your hips open by placing your elbows on your legs while hinging forward. Hold for 10–15 breaths.

Key Points

* Continue pressing your knees down with your elbows and hinging forward from the hips with each exhale.

* To reduce stress on your knees, move your feet forward. Increase the intensity of the stretch by bringing the knees closer.

* Avoid rounding your back and focus on lengthening from the hips to the crown of the head.

Modification

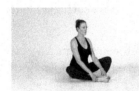

Place your feet further away from the body and sit up tall. Leave out the forward hinge movement.

■ STRADDLE SPLITS

AREAS TARGETED: Hips, back, hamstrings, calves, neck and ankles

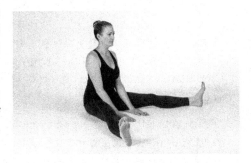

1. From Butterfly, extend the legs into Straddle and place your hands on the floor. Inhale and sit up tall, with your shoulders back and down and your chest open.

2. Exhale and walk the hands forward, keeping a straight back and pressing the backs of your knees down. Hinge forward from your hips. Practice for 10–15 breaths.

Key Points

- Keep your legs rotated outward and feet flexed as you hinge forward.
- When walking your hands forward, widen them the further you travel.
- To help widen your Straddle, hinge forward and place your hands on the insides of your legs and press them open.

Modification

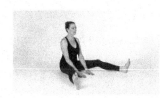

Bend your knees to take tension off the hamstrings and lower back.

◼FIGURE FOUR

AREAS TARGETED: Hips, glutes, lower back
A staple for all serious stretching routines.

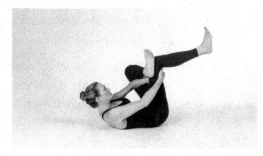

1. Lie on your back, bend your right knee, place your right foot flat on the ground and place your left ankle on top of your right thigh.

2. Reach your left arm in between your legs and your right arm around the outside. Lace your fingers together on the back of your right leg.

3. Exhale and pull your legs towards you, using your left elbow to press into your left leg to further open the stretch. The head and shoulder may come off the mat if you wish. Pump 5–10 breaths into this stretch and repeat on both sides.

Key Points

• This is a fantastic stretch for relief from intense squat, crouch and lunge training.

• The closer you place your grounded foot to your glutes, the more intense the stretch. You may extend your other leg to the sky for an extra hamstring stretch.

• Actively pull your legs closer with each exhale and sway slightly side to side to target your hip and glute muscles deeper.

Modification

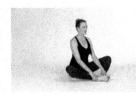

If this stretch is too tight and constricted, practice Butterfly (page 188) to loosen up your hips.

SPIDER

AREAS TARGETED: Hamstrings and calves

The Spider is a frozen Single Straight Leg Stretch (page 64) designed to expand and lengthen your hamstrings.

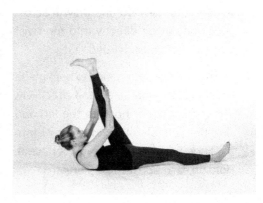

1. Lie on your back and extend your left leg to the sky. Lengthen your right leg in front of you on the floor. Grab your left leg on the ankle, calf or hamstring and lengthen further and lift your head, neck and shoulders off the mat as you exhale.

2. Inhale, bend your left knee slightly and exhale further into the stretch. Bring your nose towards your knee and flex the elevated foot with each exhale.

Key Points

- Keep your elbows pointed to the outside so you have more space to maneuver deeper into the stretch.
- Keep your hips square.
- When bringing your nose towards your knee, lift with your abdominals, not your neck and head.

Modification

Bend the leg which is extended onto the floor and place your foot flat on the ground. This will give your lower back more support in the stretch.

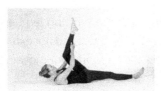 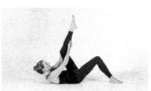

LYING SPINAL TWIST

AREAS TARGETED: Spine, back, glutes, and chest
Everyone enjoys and benefits greatly from this life-changing twist.

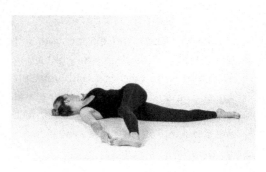

1. From Spider Stretch (page 191) either bend the top left leg and draw it across your body or go directly into the twist with your left leg extended.

2. Exhale and use your hands to help guide your leg to the floor safely and effectively. Rotate your upper body to the left and sink the your shoulder towards or into the floor. Turn your face to your left hand. Hold on each side for 10–15 breaths.

Key Points

- Continue lengthening your leg across with your exhales. Grasp your foot or ankle with the hand that's closest and pull your foot higher.

- This stretch decompresses the spine, stretches the back and glutes, and realigns the spine. It also opens the chest, calms the mind and encourages fresh blood flow to the digestive organs.

- This stretch is also a great stress reliever, both mental and physical. Move yourself out of the way of the twist and allow it to deepen with your breaths. Relax. Release. Renew.

- Add a Pretzel Twist by bending the bottom leg and holding onto it with the hand that's closest. Pull the bottom leg away from the twisting leg.

Modification

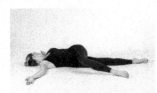

Perform this stretch with the twisting leg bent. Move into the twist with the knee into the chest and not extended upward. Use your hands to guide and support your movements.

KNEES TO CHEST

AREAS TARGETED: Lower back, glutes, quad, knees, hamstrings and spinal flexibility

Our final cooldown stretch is an ode to lower back release and regeneration.

1. Lie on your back and pull your knees to your chest. Place your hands on your knees and gently pull them and the tops of your thighs into your chest.

2. Relax your head on the mat and relax your feet and ankles. Rock your knees gently side-to-side after holding the pose for 10–15 breaths. Let go and allow the pose to release and move naturally.

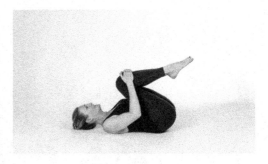

Key Points

- This stretch is a wonderful meditative experience. You will feel your low back massaging gently into the mat and the knees stretching and releasing.

- Keep your knees together while drawing them into your chest. This will increase the stretch to your quads and knees.

- For a more intense version of this stretch, bend your knees and lift your feet. Smoosh your thighs into your chest while holding your ankles. The tops of the feet point to the sky.

Modification

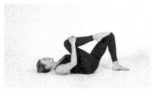

Bring one knee in at a time, with the other knee bent and your foot flat on the floor.

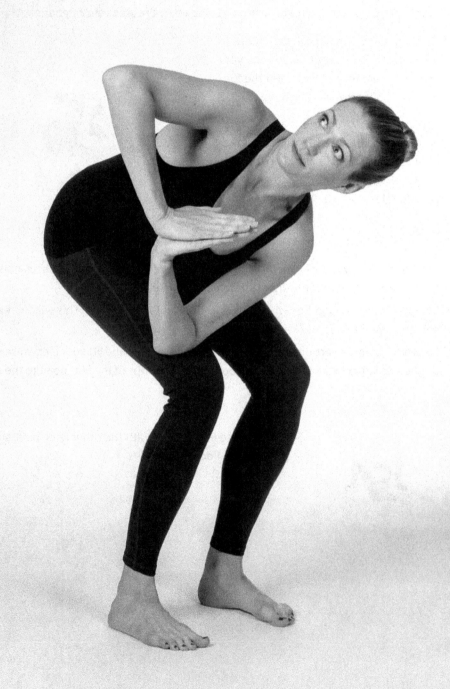

CHAPTER 8

The Flows

We now have our warm-ups, exercises, add-ons, variations, modifications, power moves, cooldown stretches . . . and much more in between. Your athletic training arsenal has grown to include hundreds of new dynamic and powerful exercises, and every single one is designed to improve your sports performance on many levels.

The challenging, diverse and unpredictable flows in this chapter allow you to create your own Pilates practice, one exercise at a time. The flows are built to accommodate athletes of all skill levels—from beginner, intermediate, and advanced to the master level of an elite athlete. Remember that your solo Pilates practice is results-driven, so use these 20 complete Pilates workouts to achieve the athletic performance results you want and need. The more time you put in, the more benefits you shall receive.

Pilates is a flowing discipline, with each exercise performed fully and completely through your range of motion before transitioning to the next. Practice (I use this word a lot—and with good reason) connecting from the end of one exercise, through the movement, into the start of the next. That is an art unto itself, and one which requires your full focus and discipline. As Joe said, "Concentrate on the correct movement each time you exercise, lest you do them improperly and thus lose all vital benefits." In other words, quality over quantity.

Do not attempt to do these flows without practicing the individual exercises presented in the previous chapters. Please also remember that Pilates should never push you to the point of getting hurt, nor be too easy as to bring no positive change.

If you're new to Pilates, start with the beginner flows and progress as your body adapts. Move to the more challenging flows only when your body and mind hunger for more of a challenge and the movements become automatic and easy. Pilates should never be mundane or boring.

For my specific workouts designed for each sport, check out the training logs in Chapter 8.

> ### You can do all these flows with Sean by visiting
> ### SeanVigueFitness.com/PilatesforAthletesBook.

1: ON-THE-GO FLOW [BEGINNER]

Never practiced Pilates before? This is the flow for you.

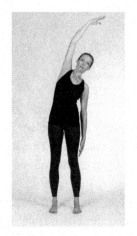 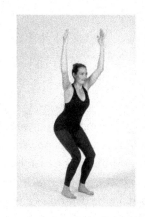 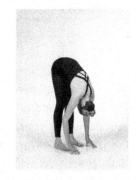

1. Standing Side Bends (10 reps)   **2.** Chair pose (5 breaths)   **3.** Forward Fold (5 breaths)

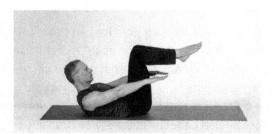

4. Modified Pilates 100

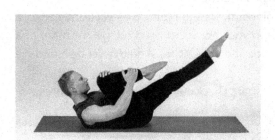 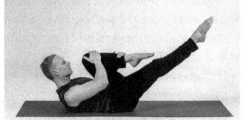

5. One Leg Stretch (10 reps)

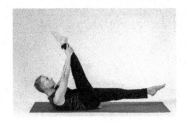
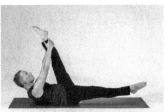

6. Single Straight Leg Stretch (10 reps)

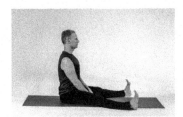
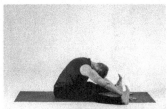

7. Spine Stretch (6 reps)

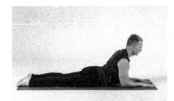
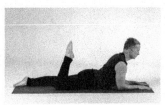
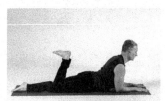

8. Saw (10 reps)

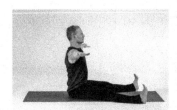
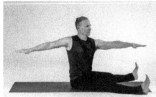

9. Single Leg Kick (10 reps)

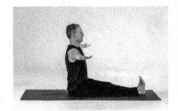
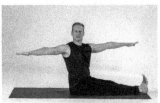
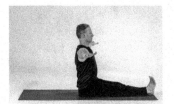

10. Spine Twist (10 reps)

2: ON-THE-GO FLOW [INTERMEDIATE]

Practice a steady rhythm of speed and control.

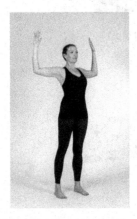

1. Standing Cactus Arms (5 reps)

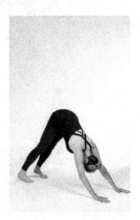

2. Downward Facing Dog with Walks (20 steps)

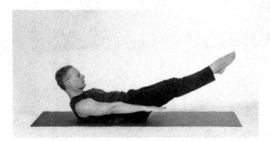

3. Pilates 100

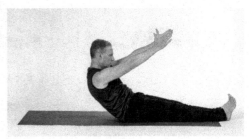

4. The Roll Up (6 reps)

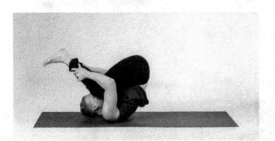

5. Rolling like a Ball (6 reps)

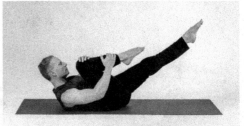

6. One Leg Stretch (14 reps)

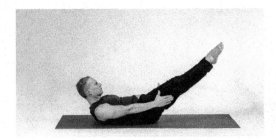

7. Double Leg Stretch (10 reps)

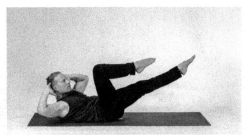

8. Crisscross (20 reps)

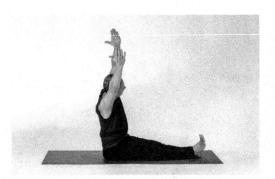

9. Seated Side-to-Side (10 reps)

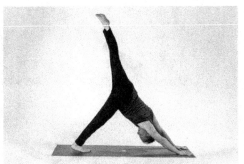

10. Downdog Leg Lifts (20 reps)

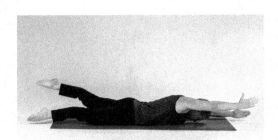

11. Swimming (10 reps)

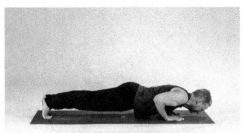

12. Push-Ups (10 reps)

3: ON-THE-GO FLOW [ADVANCED]

Challenge all your systems in a short, intense session.

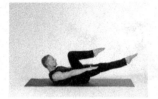 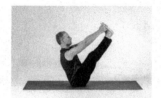 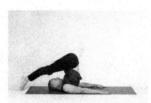

1. Single Leg Stretch 100   **2.** Roll Up to Extended Boat (6 reps)   **3.** The Roll Over (6 reps)

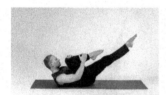 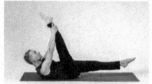 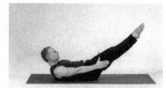

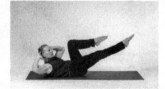 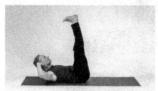

4. Big 5 Series (10 reps of each exercise)

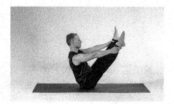 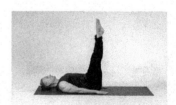

5. Open Leg Rocker (6 reps)   **6.** Corkscrew (10 circles each direction)

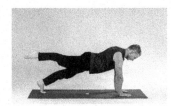

7. Leg Pull Front (10 leg lifts)

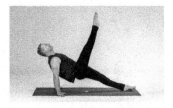

8. Leg Pull (10 kicks)

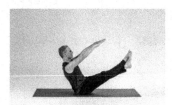

9. Pulling the Straps (10 reps)

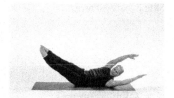

10. Superman Banana (10 reps)

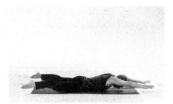

11. Boomerang (4 reps)

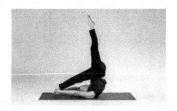

12. Control Balance (10 reps)

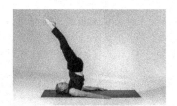

13. Jackknife (4 reps)

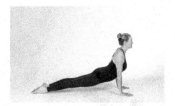

14. Upward Facing Dog (5 breaths)

4: FULL BODY WORKOUT [BEGINNER]

Once you feel solid with the beginner's on-the-go flow, turn your attention to this one which requires more stamina and concentration.

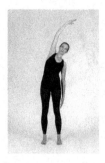

1. Side Bends (10 reps)

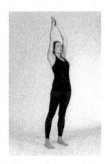

2. Backbends (5 breaths)

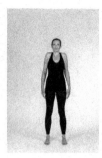

3. Shoulder Rolls (10 reps)

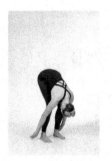

4. Flop Downs (5 reps)

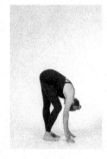

5. Forward Fold Walks (10 steps)

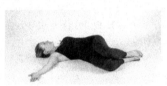

6. Windshield Wipers (10 reps)

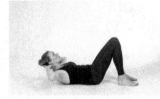

7. Chest Lifts (10 reps)

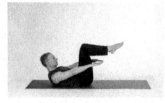

8. Modified Pilates 100

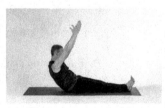

9. Half Roll Backs (6 reps)

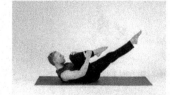

10. One Leg Stretch (10 reps)

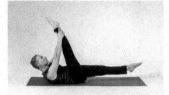

11. Single Straight Leg Stretch (10 reps)

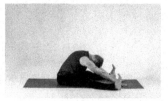

12. Spine Stretch (6 reps)

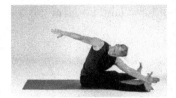

13. Saw
(10 reps)

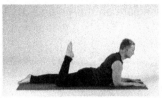

14. Single Leg Kick
(10 kicks)

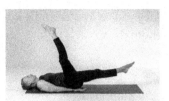

15. Scissors - Modified on
Your Back (10 reps)

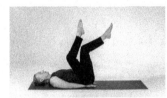

16. Bicycle - Modified on Your
Back (10 reps each direction)

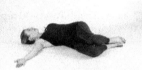

17. Windshield Wipers
(10 reps)

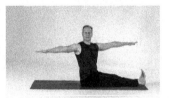

18. Spine Twist
(10 reps)

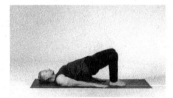

19. Shoulder Bridge
hold (5 breaths)

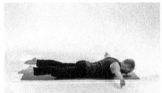

20. Pulling T-Straps
(6 reps)

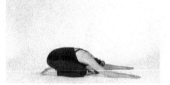

21. Child's Pose
(5 breaths)

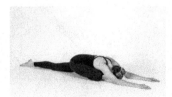

22. Pigeon
(5 breaths)

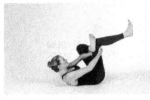

23. Figure Four
(5 breaths each side)

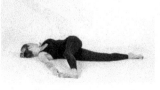

24. Lying Spinal Twist
(5 breaths on each side)

5: FULL BODY WORKOUT [INTERMEDIATE]

Once you've mastered the intermediate on the-go flow, try your hand (and body) at this full length class.

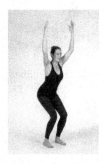

1. Chair Pose (10 breaths)

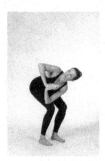

2. Chair Pose with Twists (10 reps)

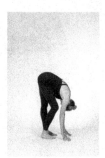

3. Forward Fold Walks (10 steps)

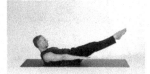

4. Pilates 100

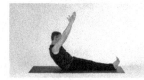

5. Half Roll Backs (6 reps)

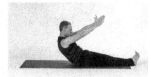

6. The Roll Up (6 reps)

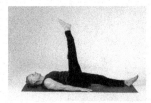

7. One Leg Circles (10 circles each direction with each leg)

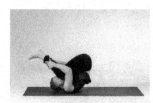

8. Rolling like a Ball (6 reps)

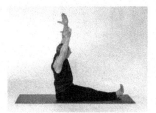

9. Seated Side-to-Side (10 reps)

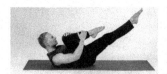
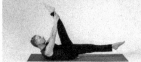
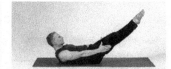

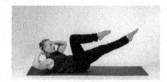
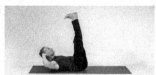

10. Big 5 Series (10 reps of each exercise)

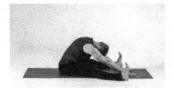

11. Spine Stretch (6 reps)

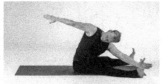

12. Saw (10 reps)

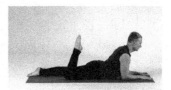

13. Single Leg Kicks (10 reps)

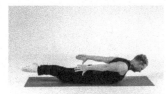

14. Double Leg Kicks
(6 reps)

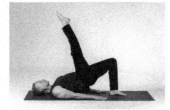

15. Shoulder Bridge
(6 reps on each leg)

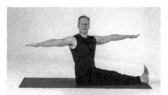

16. Spine Twist
(10 reps)

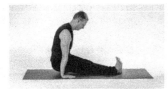

17. Tendon Stretch (10 reps)

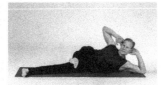

18. Side Kick (10 kicks each leg)

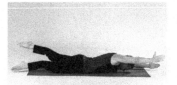

19. Swimming (10 reps)

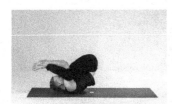

20. The Seal (6 reps)

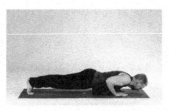

21. Push-Ups (10 reps)

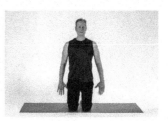

22. Chest Expansion (6 reps)

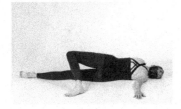

23. Scorpion
(5 breaths on each side)

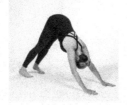

24. Downward Facing Dog
(10 breaths)

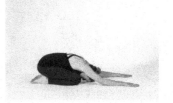

25. Child's Pose
(10 breaths)

6: FULL BODY WORKOUT [ADVANCED]

The intensity, stamina and strength needed to complete this flow will challenge your mental and physical reserves.

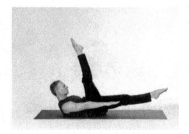

1. Scissors Pilates 100

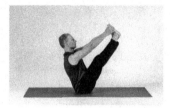

2. Roll Up to Extended Boat
(8 reps)

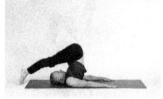

3. Roll Over
(6 reps)

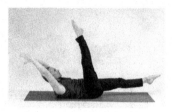

4. One Leg Circles with Arms Overhead (10 circles each direction on both sides)

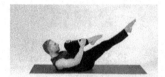

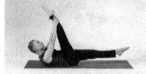

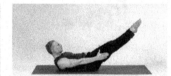

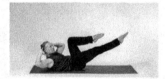

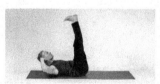

5. Big 5 Series
(10 reps of each exercise)

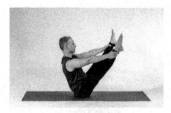

6. Open Leg Rocker with Open Close Legs on Top (6 reps)

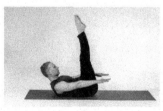

7. Corkscrew with Arms to Sides
(10 circles each direction)

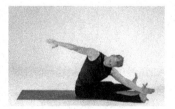

8. Saw
(10 reps)

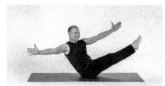

9. Boat Twists
(10 reps)

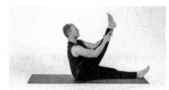

10. Tree Crunch to Hurdle Stretch
(6 reps on each side)

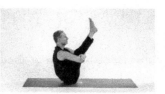

11. Extended Boat to Wrap
(6 breaths for each position)

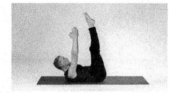

12. Backstroke (10 reps)

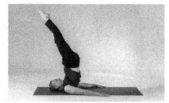

13. Jackknife (6 reps)

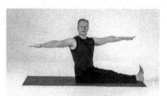

14. Spine Twist (10 reps)

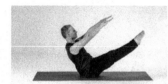

15. Teaser (6 reps)

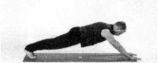

16. Elephant Planks (5 reps)

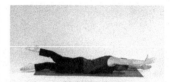

17. Swimming Fast (10 breaths)

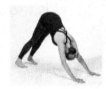

18. Downward Facing
Dog Walks (20 steps)

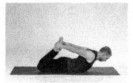

19. Rocking
(10 reps)

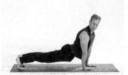

20. Snake
(6 reps each side)

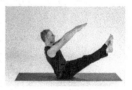

21. Boomerang
(6 reps)

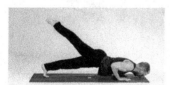

22. Push-Ups One Legged
(10 reps)

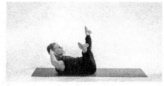

23. Straddle Crunch
(10 reps)

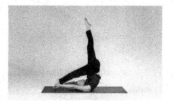

24. Control Balance
(10 reps)

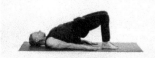

25. Bridge to Boat
(6 reps)

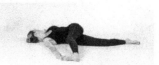

26. Lying Spinal Twist
(6 breaths each side)

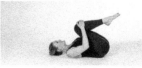

27. Knees to Chest
(10 breaths)

7: CLASSIC ABS FLOW

Turn the focus onto your abdominals with this vivid and slow burn flow.

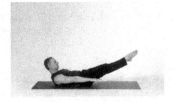

1. The Pilates 100

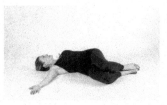

2. Windshield Wipers (10 reps)

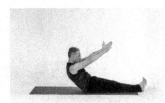

3. The Roll Up (6 reps)

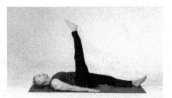

4. One Leg Circles (10 circles each direction on both sides)

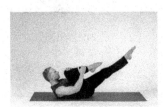
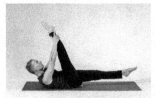
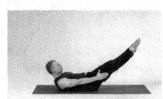
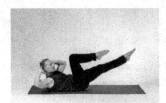
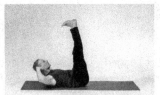

5. Big 5 Series (12 reps of each exercise)

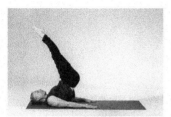

6. Corkscrew with Tail Bone
Lift (10 circles each direction
and on both sides)

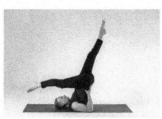

7. Scissors
(10 reps)

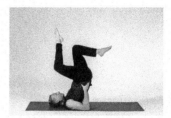

8. Bicycle
(10 circles each direction)

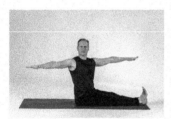

9. Spine Twist
(10 reps)

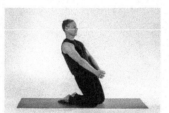

10. Camel Pulse
(10 reps)

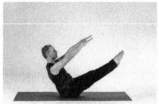

11. Teaser
(6 reps)

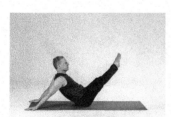

12. Hip Twist with Stretches
Arms (5 circles each direction)

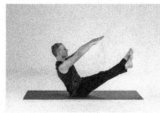

13. Boomerang
(4 reps)

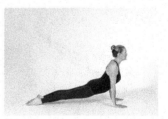

14. Cobra/Upward Facing
Dog (5 breaths)

8: CLASSIC CORE FLOW

Using exercises from the classic workout focuses, as Joseph said, "The mastery of your mind over the complete control of your body".

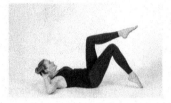

1. Toe Touches (10 reps)

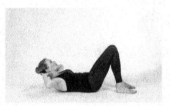

2. Chest Lifts (10 reps)

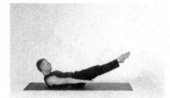

3. Pilates 100

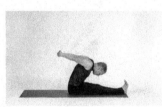

4. The Roll Up with Mudra (6 reps)

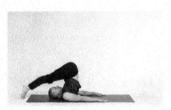

5. The Roll Over (4 reps)

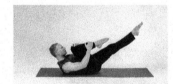

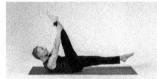

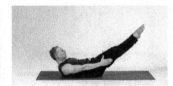

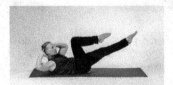

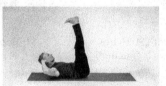

6. Big 5 Series (12 reps of each exercise)

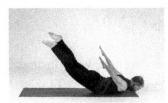

7. Swan Dive (5 reps)

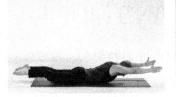

8. Double Leg Kick with Superman (6 reps)

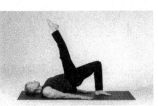

9. Shoulder Bridge (10 kicks on each side)

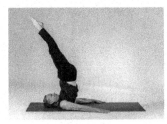

10. Jackknife (6 reps))

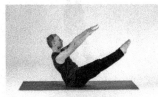

11. Teaser (6 reps)

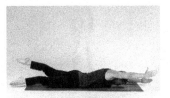

12. Swimming Fast (10 breaths)

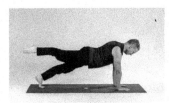

13. Leg Pull Front (10 reps)

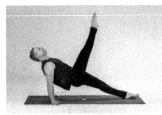

14. Leg Pull (10 kicks)

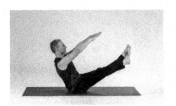

15. Boomerang (4 reps)

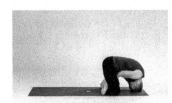

16. The Crab (4 reps)

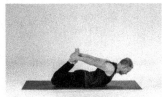

17. Rocking (10 reps)

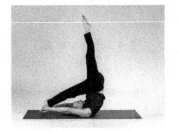

18. Control Balance (10 reps)

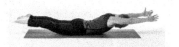

19. Push-Ups with Superman (8 reps)

9: FLEXIBILITY AND MOBILITY FLOW

Great for rehabbing and rehabilitating the body during rest days, days off or when injured.

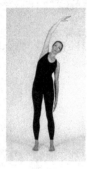

1. Side Bends
(10 reps)

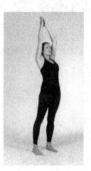

2. Backbend
(5 breaths)

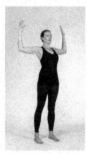

3. Cactus Arms
(5 reps)

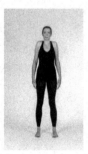

4. Shoulder Rolls
(5 reps)

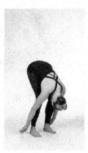

5. Flop Downs
(5 reps)

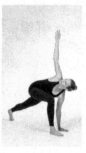

6. Lunge Twist
(5 breaths on each side)

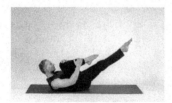

7. The One Leg Stretch
(10 reps)

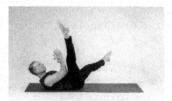

8. Single Straight Leg Stretch
with Tornados (10 reps)

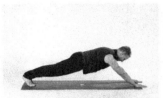

9. Elephant Planks
(5 reps)

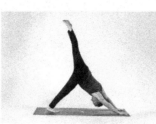

10. Downdog Leg Lifts
(20 lifts)

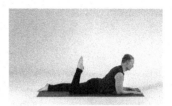

11. Single Leg Kick
(10 kicks)

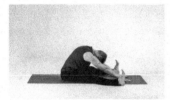

12. Spine Stretch
(6 reps)

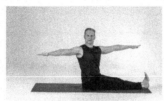

13. Spine Twist
(10 reps)

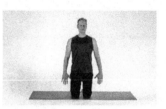

14. Chest Expansion
(6 reps)

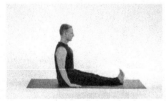

15. Rowing from the Hips
(10 reps)

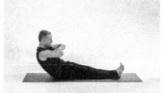

16. Rowing from Sternum
(6 reps)

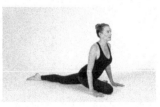

17. Proud Pigeon
(5 breaths)

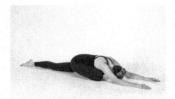

18. Pigeon
(6 breaths)

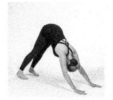

19. Downward Facing Dog Walks
(10 reps)

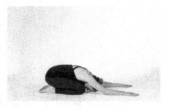

20. Child's Pose
(10 breaths)

10: MORNING PILATES FLOW

Start your day right with a positive attitude, fresh blood and oxygen flow through the body and a strong focus.

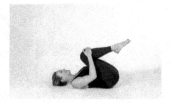

1. Knees to Chest
(5 breaths)

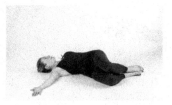

2. Windshield Wipers
(10 reps)

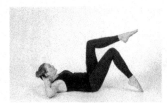

3. Toe Touches
(10 reps)

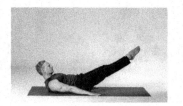

4. Coordination
(10 reps)

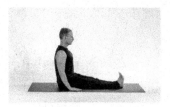

5. Rowing from the Hips
(8 reps)

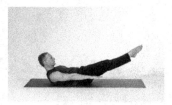

6. Pilates 100

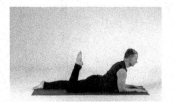

7. Single Leg Kicks
(10 reps)

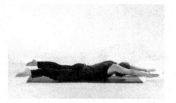

8. Pulling the Straps
(8 reps)

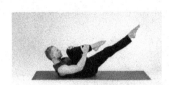
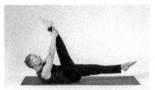
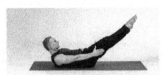
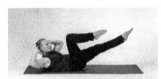
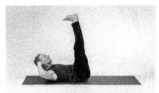

9. Big 5 Series
(10 reps of each exercise)

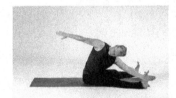
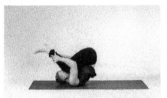
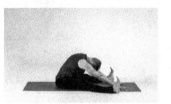

10. Saw
(10 reps)

11. Rolling like a Ball
(6 reps)

12. Spine Stretch
(6 reps)

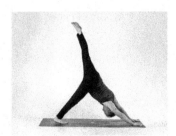
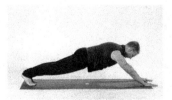

13. Downdog Leg Lifts
(10 reps)

14. Elephant Planks
(4 reps)

11: EVENING PILATES FLOW

Warm up and then cool down the body for a wonderful night of deep and renewing rest.

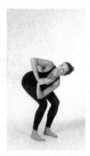

1. Chair Twists
(10 reps)

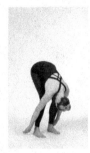

2. Slow Flop Downs
(6 reps)

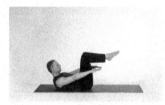

3. Pilates 100 Modified

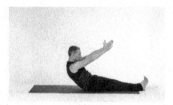

4. Half Roll Backs
(6 reps)

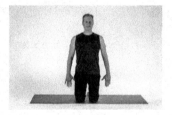

5. Chest Expansion
(6 reps)

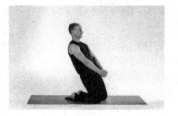

6. Camel Pulse
(5 breaths)

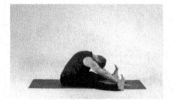

7. Spine Stretch
(6 reps)

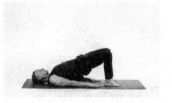

8. Bridge without Leg Lifts
(5 breaths)

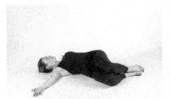

9. Windshield Wipers
(10 reps)

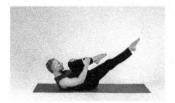

10. The One Leg Stretch
(10 reps)

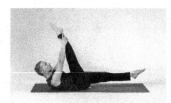

11. Single Straight Leg Stretch
(10 reps)

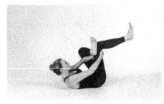

12. Figure Four
(10 breaths on each side)

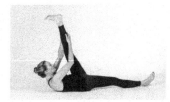

13. Spider
(8 breaths on each leg)

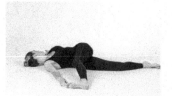

14. Lying Spinal Twist
(8 breaths on side)

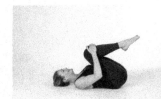

15. Knees to Chest
(10 breaths)

12: BIONIC BACK WORKOUT

Build a strong and resilient back with this full body flow.

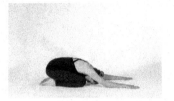

1. Child's Pose
(10 reps)

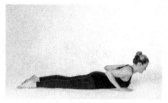

2. Cobra
(5 breaths)

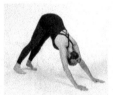

3. Downward Facing Dog with Walks
(10 steps)

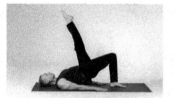

4. Shoulder Bridge
(10 leg lifts on each side)

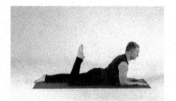

5. Single Leg Kick
(10 kicks)

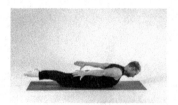

6. Double Leg Kick
(10 reps)

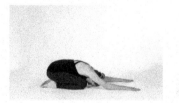

7. Child's Pose
(5 breaths)

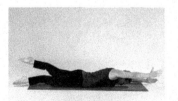

8. Swimming
(20 reps)

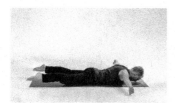

9. Pulling T-Straps
(10 reps)

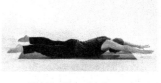

10. Pulling the Straps
(10 reps)

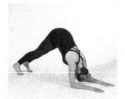

11. Dolphin
(8 breaths)

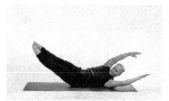

12. Superman Banana
(10 reps)

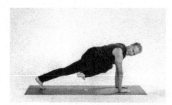

13. Spiderman Planks
(30 reps)

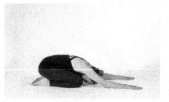

14. Child's Pose
(5 breaths)

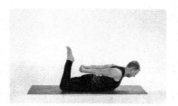

15. Rock and Pull
(10 reps)

13: ATHLETIC TRAINING FLOW

Increase your agility and strength with this comprehensive flow.

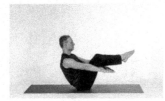

1. Boat Pilates 100

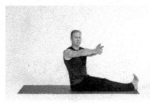

2. Roll Up Twist
(6 reps)

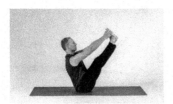

3. Rolling like a Ball to Extended Boat
(6 reps)

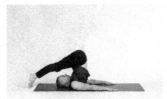

4. The Roll Over
(6 reps)

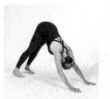

5. Downward Facing Dog
(3 breaths)

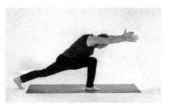

6. Lunge Crunches
(10 reps each side)

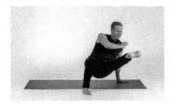

7. Kick Throughs
(20 reps)

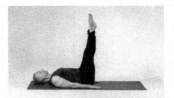

8. Corkscrew
(10 circles each direction)

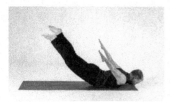

9. Swan Dive
(6 reps)

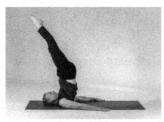

10. Jackknife
(6 reps)

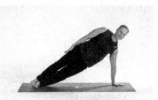

11. Star
(6 reps)

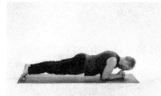

12. Pilates Planks
(10 reps)

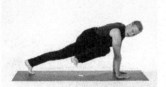

13. Spider Man Burpees
(5–10 reps)

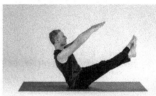

14. Boomerang
(4 reps)

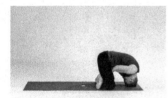

15. The Crab
(6 reps)

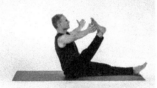

16. Tree Crunch Leg to Side
(6 reps each side)

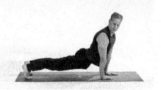

17. Snake
(3 reps on each side)

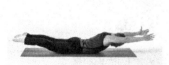

18. Superman to Teaser
(5 reps)

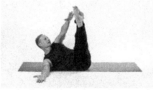

19. Pendulum with Reach
(10 reps)

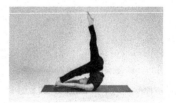

20. Control Balance
(10 reps)

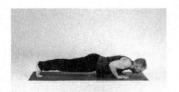

21. Push-Ups
(10 sets of 1–5 reps)

14: REHAB PILATES FLOW

Focus on flexibility, stretching and increased oxygen uptake.

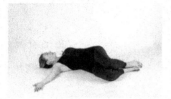

1. Windshield Wipers
(10 reps)

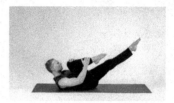

2. The One Leg Stretch
(10 reps)

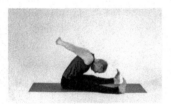

3. Spine Stretch with Mudra
(6 reps)

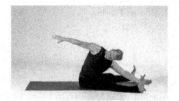

4. Saw
(10 reps)

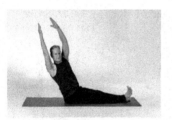

5. Seated Twist and Drop
(10 reps)

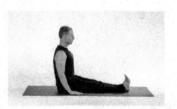

6. Rowing from the Hips
(6 reps)

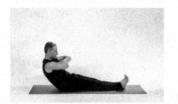

7. Rowing from the Sternum
(6 reps)

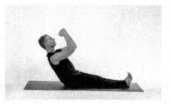

8. Rowing 90 Degrees
(6 reps)

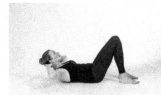

9. Chest Lift
(6 reps)

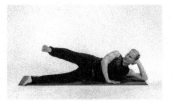

10. Side Leg Circles
(10 reps on both sides)

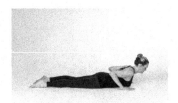

11. Cobra
(5 breaths)

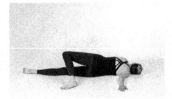

12. Scorpion
(6 breaths on each side)

13. Pyramid
(6 breaths each side)

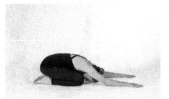

14. Child's Pose (10 breaths)

15: PRE-WORKOUT FLOW

These dynamic exercises prepare your body for your sports-specific workouts.

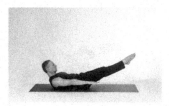

1. Pilates 100

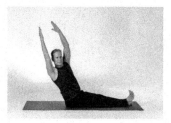

2. Seated Twist and Drop
(6 reps)

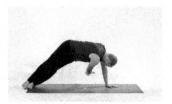

3. Side Plank Thread the Needle
(10 reps)

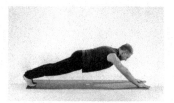

4. Walk Out Planks
(6 reps)

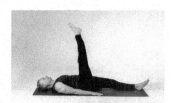

5. One Leg Circles
(10 circles in each direction, both sides)

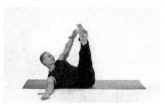

6. Pendulum with Reach
(10 reps)

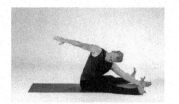

7. Saw
(10 reps)

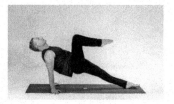

8. Leg Pull with Mountain Climbers
(10 reps)

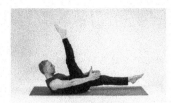

9. Single Straight Leg Stretch with
Arms to Sides (10 reps)

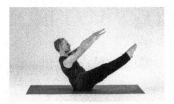

10. Teaser
(6 reps)

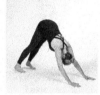

11. Downward Facing Dog
with Walks (20 steps)

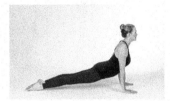

12. Upward Facing Dog
(5 breaths)

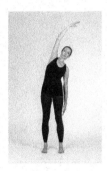

13. Side Bends
(10 reps)

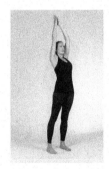

14. Backbend
(5 breaths)

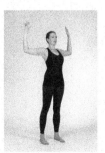

15. Cactus Arms
(5 reps)

16: POST-WORKOUT PILATES FLOW

This is an invigorating cooldown flow for even the most strenuous workouts.

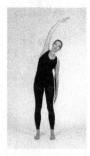

1. Side Bends
(10 reps)

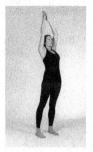

2. Backbend
(5 breaths)

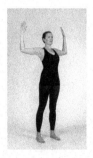

3. Cactus Arms
(5 reps)

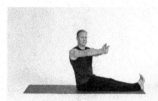

4. Roll Up with Twist
(6 reps)

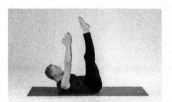

5. Backstroke
(10 reps)

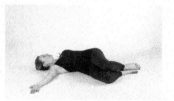

6. Windshield Wipers
(10 reps)

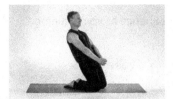

7. Camel Pulse
(6 breaths)

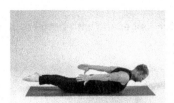

8. Double Leg Kick
(6 reps)

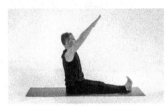

9. Rowing from the Chest
(6 reps)

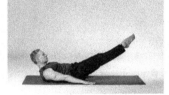

10. Coordination
(10 reps)

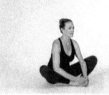

11. Butterfly
(8 breaths)

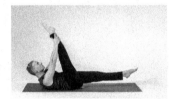

12. Single Straight Leg Stretch
(10 slow reps)

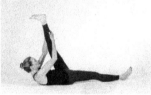

13. Spider
(6 breaths for each leg)

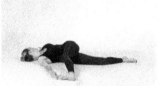

14. Lying Spinal Twist
(6 breaths each side)

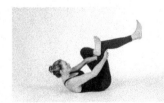

15. Figure Four
(6 breaths each side)

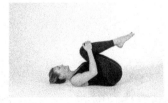

16. Knees to Chest
(10 breaths)

17: PILATES FOR RUNNERS FLOW

Run faster, longer and with better form by adding this sequence to your training.

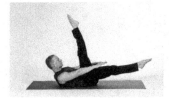

1. Scissors Pilates 100

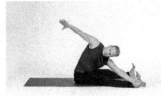

2. Roll Up Saw
(6 reps)

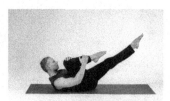

3. One Leg Stretch
(10 reps)

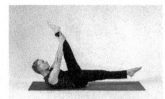

4. Single Straight Leg Stretch
(10 reps)

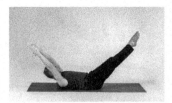

5. Double Leg Stretch with Arms
Reaching Overhead
(10 reps)

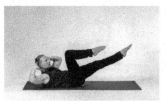

6. Crisscross
(20 reps)

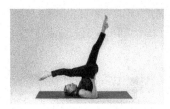

7. Scissors
(10 reps)

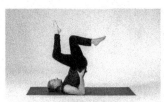

8. Bicycle
(10 reps)

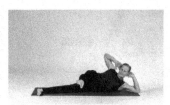

9. Side Kicks
(10 reps each side)

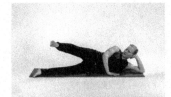

10. Side Leg Circles
(10 reps on both sides)

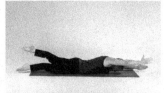

11. Swimming Fast
(10 breaths)

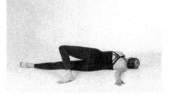

12. Scorpion - Active
(10 reps side-to-side)

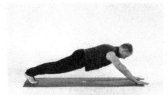

13. Elephant Planks
(5 reps)

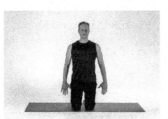

14. Chest Expansion
(6 reps)

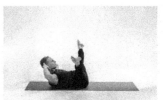

15. Straddle Crunch
(10 reps)

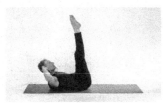

16. Reverse Straddle Crunch
(10 reps)

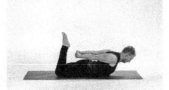

17. Rock and Pull
(6 reps)

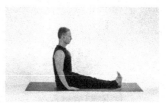

18. Rowing from the Hips
(10 reps)

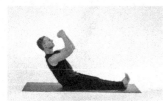

19. Rowing 90 Degrees
(6 reps)

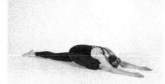

20. Pigeon
(6 breaths each side)

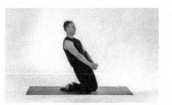

21. Camel Pulse
(6 breaths)

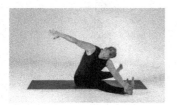

22. Straddle Saw
(10 breaths)

18: PILATES FOR ENDURANCE FLOW

Work on performing this flow with minimum rest in between exercises and more speed (while always maintaining proper form) to expand your endurance and cardiopulmonary potential.

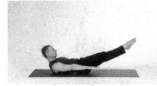

1. Pilates 100

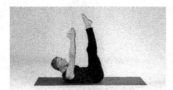

2. Backstroke
(10 reps)

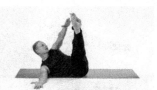

3. Pendulum with Reach
(10 reps)

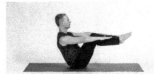

4. Roll Up to Boat
(6 reps)

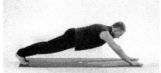

5. Walk out Planks
(10 reps)

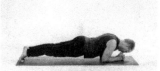

6. Pilates Planks
(10 reps)

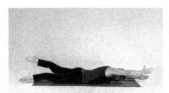

7. Swimming Fast
(10 breaths)

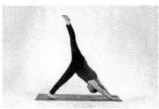

8. Down Dog with Leg Lifts
(20 reps)

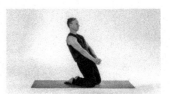

9. Camel Pulse
(10 reps)

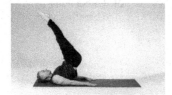

10. Corkscrew with Tail Bone Lift
(10 circles each direction)

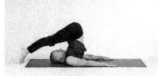

11. Roll Over
(6 reps)

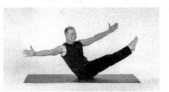

12. Boat Twists
(10 reps))

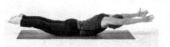

13. Superman Burpees
(5–10 reps)

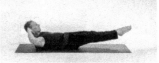

14. Oval Crunches
(10 reps)

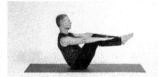

15. Roll Up to Boat
(6 reps)

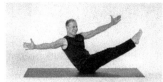

16. Boat Twists
(10 reps)`

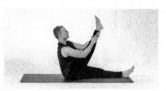

17. Tree Crunch to Hurdle Stretch
(6 reps each side)

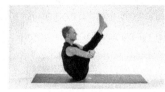

18. Extended Boat to Wrap
(10 breaths total)

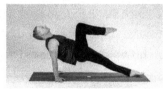

19. Leg Pull with Mountain
Climbers (20 reps)

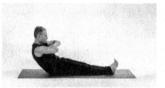

20. Rowing from
the Sternum (6 reps)

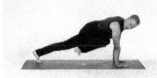

21. Spider Man Burpees
(5–10 reps)

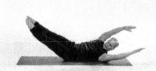

22. Superman Banana
(10 reps)

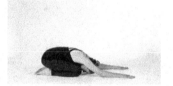

23. Child's Pose
(6 breaths)

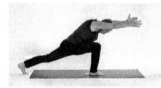

24. Lunge Crunches
(10 reps each side)

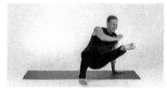

25. Kick Throughs
(20 reps)

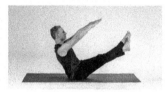

26. Boomerang
(6 reps)

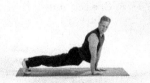

27. Snake
(4 reps each side)

28. Pyramid
(8 breaths each side)

29. Downward Facing Dog
(10 breaths)

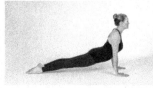

30. Cobra/Upward Facing Dog
(6 breaths)

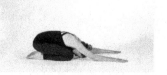

31. Child's Pose
(10 breaths)

19: CLASSIC PILATES WORKOUT

I have done this specific workout at least 30 times in preparation for writing this book and it has persistently challenged, invigorated and inspired me. First appearing in his fitness manifesto, Return to Life through Contrology, Joseph Pilates designed this original sequence of 34 movements as a complete, full body workout to enhance all aspects of your physical and mental health. I can say from experience that it indeed does enhance my mental and physical abilities. Performing this workout is like stepping back in time to when Joseph first opened his studio in New York and began his fitness revolution. The exercises have withstood the test of time, as their genius and effectiveness are more fully realized each time someone rolls out their mat and decides to spend some quality time with Joseph's movement masterpiece. (Note that I did not include the Neck Pull exercise, as I find it very uncomfortable.)

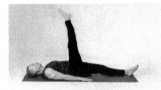
1. Pilates 100

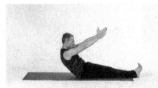
2. The Roll Up
(6 reps)

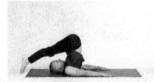
3. The Roll Over
(4 reps)

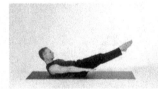
4. One Leg Circle (10 circles each direction on both sides)

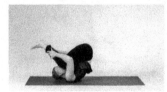
5. Rolling like a Ball
(6 reps)

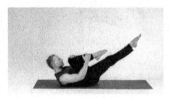
6. One Leg Stretch
(10 reps)

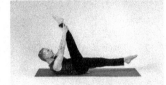
7. Single Straight Leg Stretch
(10 reps)

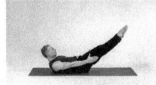
8. Double Leg Stretch
(10 reps)

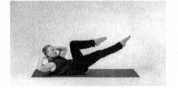
9. Crisscross
(20 reps)

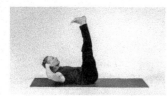

10. Double Straight Leg Stretch
(10 reps)

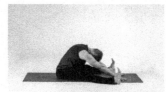

11. Spine Stretch
(6 reps)

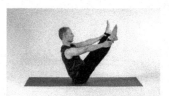

12. Open Leg Rocker
(6 reps)

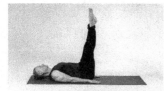

13. Corkscrew (10 circles each
direction on both sides)

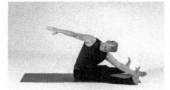

14. Saw
(10 reps)

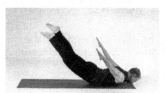

15. Swan Dive
(6 reps)`

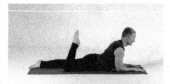

16. Single Leg Kick
(10 reps)

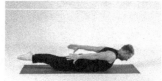

17. Double Leg Kick
(8 reps)

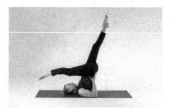

18. Scissors
(10 reps)

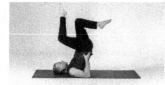

19. Bicycle (10 revolutions
each direction)

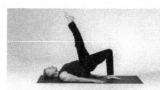

20. Shoulder Bridge
(10 leg lifts on each side)

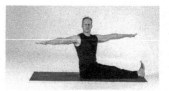

21. Spine Twist
(10 reps)

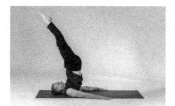

22. Jackknife
(5 reps)

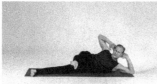

23. Side Kick
(10 kicks)

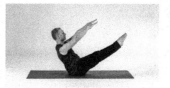

24. Teaser
(6 reps)

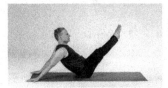

25. Hip Twist with Stretched Arms (5 circles each direction)

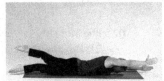

26. Swimming (10 reps)

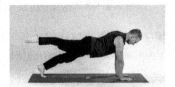

27. Leg Pull Front (10 reps)

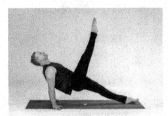

28. Leg Pull (10 kicks))

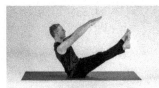

29. Boomerang (5 reps)

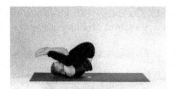

30. The Seal (6 reps)

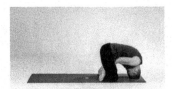

31. The Crab (6 reps)

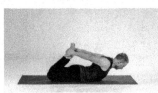

32. Rocking (10 reps

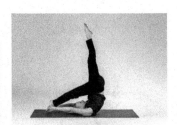

33. Control Balance (10 reps)

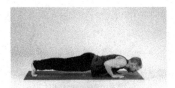

34. Push-Ups (10 reps)

20: OFFICIAL PILATES FOR OPTIMUM ATHLETIC PERFORMANCE WORKOUT

Here it is! This is the ultimate Pilates/core workout for athletes of all sports. Your Pilates goal is to complete this workout from beginning to end with minimal breaks and using only the best form, control, precision and focus. When you master this flow, I will gladly add revisions to this book with new workouts, flows and challenges.

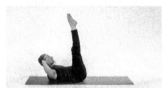

1. Single Leg Stretch 100

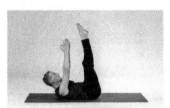

2. Backstroke
(10 reps)

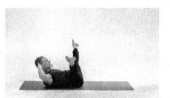

3. Straddle Crunch
(10 reps)

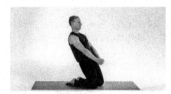

4. Reverse Straddle Crunch
(10 reps)

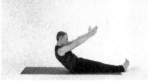

5. The Roll Up
(6 reps)

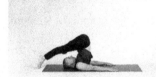

6. The Roll Over
(4 reps)

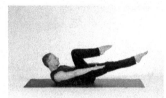

7. Camel Pulse
(10 reps)

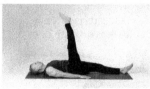

8. One Leg Circle (10 circles each direction on both sides)

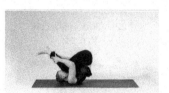

9. Rolling like a Ball
(6 reps)

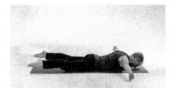

10. Pulling T-Straps
(10 reps)

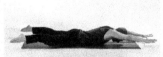

11. Pulling the Straps
(10 reps)

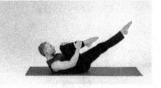

12. One Leg Stretch
(10 reps)

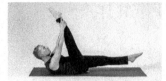

13. Single Straight Leg
Stretch (10 reps)

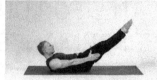

14. Double Leg Stretch
(10 reps)

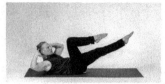

15. Criss Cross
(20 reps)

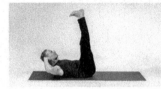

16. Double Straight Leg Stretch
(10 reps)`

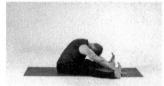

17. Spine Stretch
(6 reps)

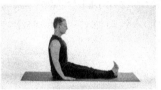

18. Rowing from the Hips
(6 reps)

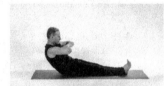

19. Rowing from the Sternum
(6 reps)

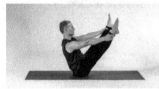

20. Open Leg Rocker
(6 reps)

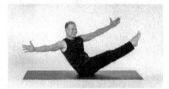

21. Boat Twist
(10 reps)

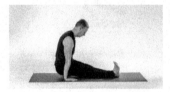

22. Tendon Stretch
(6 reps)

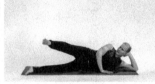

23. Side Leg Circles
(10 reps on both sides)

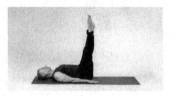

24. Corkscrew (10 circles each
direction on both sides)

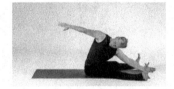

25. Saw (10 reps)

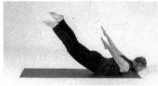

26. Swan Dive (6 reps)

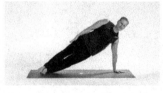

27. Star (6 reps on each side)

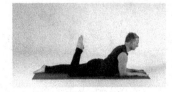

28. Single Leg Kick (10 reps)

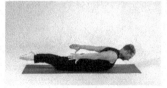

29. Double Leg Kick (8 reps)

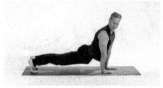

30. Snake (4 reps on each side)

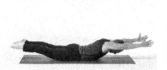

31. Superman to Boat Teaser
(2 reps on each side)

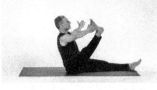

32. Tree Crunch Legs to
Side (4 reps on each side)

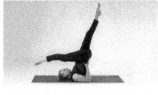

33. Scissors
(10 reps)

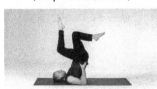

34. Bicycle (10 revolutions
each direction)`

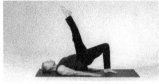

35. Shoulder Bridge
(10 leg lifts on each side)

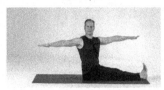

36. Spine Twist
(10 reps)

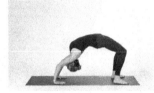

37. Wheel Pose
(hold for 5 breaths)

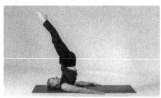

38. Jackknife
(5 reps)

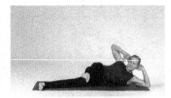

39. Side Kick
(10 kicks)

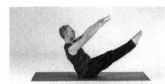

40. Teaser
(6 reps)

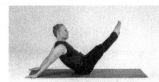

41. Hip Twist with Stretched
Arms (5 circles each direction)

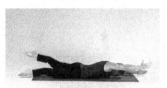

42. Swimming
(10 reps)

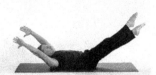

43. Reverse Swimming
(do for 5 breaths)

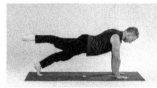

44. Leg Pull Front
(10 reps)

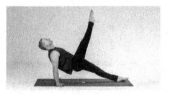

45. Leg Pull
(10 kicks)

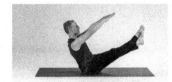

46. Boomerang
(5 reps)

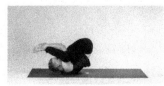

47. The Seal
(6 reps)

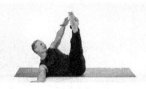

48. Pendulum with Reach
(10 reps)

237

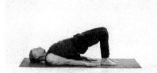

49. Bridge to Boat
(6 reps)`

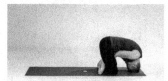

50. The Crab
(6 reps)

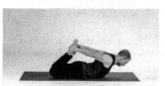

51. Rocking
(10 reps)

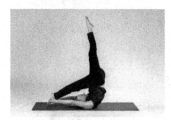

52. Control Balance
(10 reps)

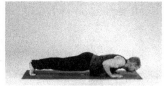

53. Push-Ups
(10 reps)

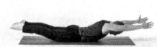

54. Superman Burpees
(5 reps)

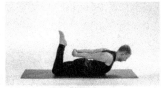

55. Rock and Pull
(6 reps)

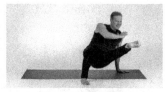

56. Kick Throughs
(20 reps)

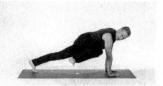

57. Spider Man Burpees
(6 reps)

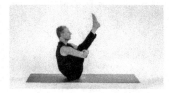

58. Extended Boat to Wrap
(hold for 10 breaths)

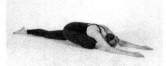

59. Pigeon
(hold for 10 breaths)

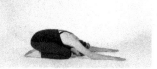

60. Child's Pose
(hold for 10 breaths)

CHAPTER 9

Sports-Specific Training Logs

The Training Logs in this chapter are designed to help you begin practicing and adding Pilates to your training in the shortest amount of time.

In each of the 15 logs, you will find:

1. A brief overview about the demands of the sport
2. How regular Pilates training will enhance your abilities
3. And a sport-specific Pilates workout flow to get you on the mat and flowing quickly

Study and practice each exercise individually before diving into the workout. Remember that hard work, precision and impeccable form are hallmarks of the Pilates mat method and are never to be taken lightly. Read, study and practice each one before moving onto the next exercise in the flow. Once you have a firm grasp on each one, only then is it time to tackle the full workout.

I have also added a few "extra credit" exercises for each sport, which can be practiced and plugged into the flow as you wish. In my experience, every exercise, stretch and flow in this book—when performed properly—will produce impressive results in a short amount of time . . . with regular practice and discipline, of course.

AMERICAN FOOTBALL/RUGBY

"Even more remarkable than his dynamic play this season is the fact that [Antonio] Brown doesn't lift weights in the off-season. Instead, he incorporates Pilates workouts into his training. They have enhanced his core strength, developed explosive power in his hips and glutes, and created muscle balance through strengthening and alignment."

—Zac Clark, stack.com

Pilates teaches athletes to move smarter, not harder. It's the nuances of a play which define your success or failure in American football and rugby, where split second changes of movement to avoid a tackle, and gauging the height, speed and arrival time of a thrown football to effectively navigate around and through blockers are commonplace. Pilates teaches immediate body control and efficiency of movement to let you effectively sustain the least amount of hits, collisions and joint wear and tear, teaching your body better ways to rebalance itself while building more power—even when you are off balance.

Football and Rugby are brutal sports. They are defined by hard hits, devastating tackles and a relentless need for constant speed and power. There are no consistent straight lines of movement, which is why we train through all angles and planes of movement. Rotation, folding forward and back (flexion and extension) and side bends (right lateral flexion and left lateral flexion) are practiced and reinforced in Pilates. Pilates also builds hamstring and back flexibility for reduced stress on the body and more resistance to injury. Your muscles will mobilize better as your joints move freely and safely.

Finally, the Pilates focus on "mind over body" helps during peak season (and through grueling practices) when risk of injury is highest. Reinforcing proper alignment, posture and deep, energy-giving breath gives a football player the stamina and vision to compete at their highest level in practice, throughout the season and into the playoffs.

AMERICAN FOOTBALL/RUGBY
PILATES CONDITIONING WORKOUT

1. **Chair with Twist**
2. **Pilates 100**
3. **The Big 5 Series**
4. **Double Leg Kick**
5. **Shoulder Bridge**
6. **Leg Pull Front**
7. **Push-Ups**
8. **Pilates Planks**
9. **Pulling the Straps**
10. **Superman Burpees**

⚾ BASEBALL

"What I noticed from Pilates last year was that I have much better control of my body. I repeat my delivery consistently. My balance is much improved. And the mental and physical toughness Pilates requires to complete movements the correct way has directly helped me on the mound."

—Jake Arrieta

When baseball season comes upon us, it brings with it the warm weather, longer days . . . the smell of grilling food and the sound of a bat crack as the crowd roars. It's a wonderful time of the year, and that goes for the players, too . . . so long as they are using Pilates training for their athletic baseball conditioning.

Baseball movements bring the athlete to the very edge of their movement range (the swing through of the bat, the follow through on the pitch, sprinting to first base, diving for the ball or a base, and jumping to our full height to catch a line drive). All of which the mobility and flexibility training of Pilates will assist and expand; the dynamic strengthening and stretching nature of Pilates exercises trains the body to move to its threshold with ease and precision. The progressive challenge of Pilates workouts will expand your body's physical and mental limits.

The Pilates focus on core strength and stability creates harder hitters and more accurate pitchers. Batters needs a steady supply of rotational force and power when stepping up to the plate for maximum hitting distance and accuracy, and pitchers need consistent core power and flexibility through the glutes and lower back to throw with speed, accuracy and efficiency. As in other sports where only the dominant side is used (as when swinging, pitching and throwing), balance must be brought to the body with Pilates. If both sides are not strengthened and stretched, massive imbalances will sweep through the body and open it to all sorts of debilitating injuries. Pilates keeps the core and body supple, flexible and resilient for consistent play all the way through the 162-game season, into the playoffs and onward into the World Series!

BASEBALL PILATES CONDITIONING WORKOUT

1. Scorpion
2. The Roll Up Twist
3. One Leg Circles
4. Corkscrew
5. Saw
6. Swan Dive
7. Scissors
8. Swimming
9. Tree Crunch to Hurdle Stretch
10. Side Plank Thread the Needle

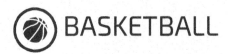 BASKETBALL

"I really felt the Pilates loosen up my muscles. I recall making a move, and the basketball ended up on my foot and I almost did a split on the ball. Normally, that's a groin pull, but I bounced back."

—Dwayne Wade

Pilates is essential for optimum basketball conditioning. Basketball consists of running, passing, jumping and shooting, causing tight hips and hamstrings, sore lower backs and injured ankles. It is one of the most physically demanding sports, with quick changes of direction requiring core stability, body control and precision of movement. When setting up for a jump shot, players must stop on a dime, rotate and jump, all while gauging the height, speed and distance the ball must travel to the basket. When passing on the run, force must be applied with quickness and accuracy in a split second. Focus and a clear mind are essential.

Practicing Pilates teaches players how to move from their core outward, maintaining proper alignment up and down the court. Building core stability with Pilates improves the efficiency of your movement, creating a quicker and more controlled athlete. This will increase your jumping, running and shooting skills while decreasing your risk of injury. Flexibility training will also assist with your body's agility when dribbling and posting up for shots.

BASKETBALL PILATES CONDITIONING WORKOUT

1. Downward Facing Dog
2. Single Leg Stretch 100
3. One Leg Circle
4. Spine Stretch
5. Corkscrew
6. Saw
7. Double Leg Kick
8. Swimming
9. Tree Crunch to Hurdle Stretch
10. Push-Ups

CYCLING

When I teach spinning classes (indoor cycling), I emphasize a tall, balanced posture in the saddle. Bicycling is low impact and easy on the knees, but the repetitive pedaling revolutions over time will bring compression and tightness to the hips and lower back. Your posture is also kept in a slightly forward position pushing through the quads, which constricts the hip flexors. Riders must stretch and open their hips, hamstrings and back to balance out this tightness, which can become a serious issue if not addressed and can lead to pain and soreness

The upper body postural work of Pilates is imperative to help lift and expand the chest and shoulders, which tend to sink over long rides. Pilates balance and control comes in handy for riders who favor uneven terrains and trails, such as mountain bikers or anyone who prefers going off road. Let a strong core be your center and guide through all terrains.

The Side Leg series is particularly helpful with pedal strength and power by building not just the larger muscles but the neglected supporting muscles of the legs, while including extra hip mobility. Adding powerful, focused Pilates breath awareness to your ride will also keep you tall, balanced and filled with extra endurance and focus.

According to Bicycle.com: "It's especially important for cyclists to focus on strengthening their back and hip stability," Rachel Pisken, a certified Pilates instructor says. "Pilates can help cyclists learn how to properly engage and activate the core, back, and hips to maintain strong form on the bike and prevent injury."

CYCLING PILATES CONDITIONING WORKOUT

1. Cobra/Updog
2. Single Leg Stretch 100
3. Roll Up Saw
4. The Roll Over with Open/Close Legs
5. The Big 5 Series
6. Corkscrew
7. Bicycle (of course)
8. Leg Pull
9. Camel Pulse
10. Rock and Pull

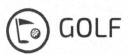 # GOLF

"Tiger [Woods] is religious about fitness and incorporates Pilates into his exercise regime. Now Pilates has become recognized in golf as a must to improve your game and prolong your career."

—FORRESTPILATES.COM

If you're a golfer and have not had the opportunity to add Pilates to your training, you are in for a HUGE treat! Pilates provides spectacular core stability, hip and low back flexibility and body control to increase the efficiency of your backswing and follow through. Golf demands that a smooth transfer of force be applied from the backswing through to the front swing, with a strong, balanced core providing an anchor against the movement. Steady rotational force is needed to ensure a strong and accurate shot, regardless of the terrain of the course.

Golf also predominantly favors one side of the body, causing overuse injuries and the weakening of underused muscles and creating imbalances which hinder your abilities on the links. For balanced alignment and posture, the golfer needs to train both sides—regardless of which side they favor. If only one side is trained and allowed to flourish, the opposite side's muscles will atrophy, causing severe imbalances and pain which will derail your golf game.

Golf is also a quiet game with a calmness to its movements. The ability to breathe effectively into your backswing (inhale) and front swing (exhale) will enhance your follow through, precision and control. Whether it's a long drive, medium show or a game-winning putt, your Pilates training will give you balance, control, flexibility, power, focus and proper breath support.

GOLF PILATES CONDITIONING WORKOUT

1. **Lunge with Twist**
2. **Windshield Wipers**
3. **Pilates 100**
4. **Single Straight Leg Stretch**
5. **Criss Cross**
6. **Saw**
7. **Shoulder Bridge**
8. **Spine Twist**
9. **Boat Twists**
10. **Pendulum with Reach**

⊘ HOCKEY

"I take it seriously. It helps to heal my mind. It's a great way to be strong and stay focused at the same time. I wish I knew Pilates before. I feel very good."
—PHILLIP DANAULT

Hockey is my favorite sport, and one I played for 10 years on the frozen lakes, ponds and rinks of snow in arctic Wisconsin. It's a non-stop cardiovascular sport and requires a *lot* of stamina and breath control, with players on the ice for many minutes without a whistle blow. Proper, deep diaphragm breathing is essential to fuel the many quick bursts of speed, back-and-forth plays (which seem to never end) and constant directional changes the game of hockey demands. The deep Pilates breathing practice will increase your respiratory efficiency and give you that extra bit of energy to carry you through, all while increasing the power of your wrist shots, slap shots and passing game thanks to the stronger breath (and core) behind them.

Your shots and passes will also have much more speed and accuracy due to a flexible and strong core. While hockey uses the forehand and backhand, it's natural to assume your forehand will always have more strength. Pilates helps cultivate a strong backhand too, which will be quite sufficient on the ice.

Oh, and do you like to check? A stronger center of balance and strength will increase the power of your checks while also keeping you gliding quickly across the ice.

The muscular imbalances which many hockey players face due to dominant side play can be corrected with regular Pilates practice emphasizing flexibility and mobility in the hips and trunk. Groin injuries are very common on the ice. Your key to injury prevention hockey is a pliable and flexible body.

And one last thing: hockey players find themselves predominantly in a crouched, hinged forward position, which causes poor postural and alignment issues. Pilates focuses on stretching and strengthening the entire back from the neck directly down to the bottom of the spine.

HOCKEY PILATES
CONDITIONING WORKOUT

1. **Lunge with Twist**
2. **Pilates 100**
3. **The Roll Up Twist**
4. **One Leg Circles**
5. **Corkscrew**
6. **Single Leg Kick**
7. **Swimming fast**
8. **Seated Twist and Drop**
9. **Pulling the Straps**
10. **Rowing Series**

⊗ LACROSSE

I received a lot of requests to include lacrosse after leaving it out of my last book *Power Yoga for Athletes*. Lacrosse has enjoyed a huge boom in popularity the past 10 years and shows no signs of slowing down. Adding Pilates to your current lacrosse conditioning program will yield huge results in speed, strength, agility and rotational power.

Lacrosse players sprint and stop continually, placing a large demand on their cardio, strength and endurance. Learning how to breathe into your deep abdominal muscles is necessary to sustain and support this level of cardiovascular movement. Better breath awareness ensures you will not make the mistake of holding your breath while playing, becoming lightheaded, weak and dizzy, and even passing out.

How are the speed and accuracy of your lacrosse shots? The strong rotational force needed for powerful shots begins in the legs and travels through the hips and the core, before arriving at the shoulders and arms. The core (powerhouse) is the center of your power, remember? Pilates trains the core so rotational force is balanced and strong. Using your Pilates training, you can bring strength, control, flexibility and a high level of functional movement to your playing ability.

LACROSSE PILATES CONDITIONING WORKOUT

1. Pigeon
2. Scissors 100
3. The Big 5 Series
4. Spine Stretch Mudra
5. Saw
6. Double Leg Kick
7. Hip Twist with Stretched Arms
8. Leg Pull Front
9. Push Ups with Superman
10. Pilates Planks with One Leg

MARTIAL ARTS

The man himself, Joseph Pilates, studied martial arts and boxing and even went to England in 1912 to study as a boxer in London. While living in London, he trained the English police in self-defense, and was well-respected in the martial arts community for training self-defense before it was popular in America.

Tae Kwando, kung fu, Jiujitsu, kickboxing, judo, karate, grappling . . . whether your style involves punching, kicking, performing takedowns, grappling or moving quickly to avoid an attack, a martial artist needs proper body control, awareness and explosive speed. Pilates teaches the martial artist to train from the core outward into the arms and legs, to better radiate strength into their punches and kicks. Having a strong core helps anchor powerful, accurate kicks and punches, and assists in controlling your opponent during groundwork. A strong center also assists in helping you move with more precision and fluidity, shifting from one position to the next with minimal effort and maximum effectiveness.

When doing kicks, punches, takedowns and grappling, if the spine is not flexible it will increase your chance of injury and hinder your abilities. Pilates stretches and decompresses the spine to increase spinal function and flexibility, keeping your body lengthened and flexible for optimum performance on the mat.

The Pilates method is also meticulous (almost to the point of insanity) when it comes to good form, flow and precision. The extra Pilates you bring into your martial arts training will smooth out the way you move, breathe, react, attack, adapt and focus. You will also build integrated strength without wear and tear on your joints, spine and posture. The Pilates focus on deep, rhythmic breathing will help increase stamina and endurance by keeping your system well supplied with oxygen.

MARTIAL ARTS PILATES CONDITIONING WORKOUT

1. Downward Facing Dog with Walks
2. Boat 100
3. The Roll Up Twist
4. The Roll Over
5. The Big 5 Series
6. Open Leg Rocker
7. Jackknife
8. Boomerang
9. One Legged Push Ups
10. Bridge to Boat

RUNNING

I enjoy trail running here in the Colorado Rockies; it's fun, challenging and unpredictable, with everchanging terrain and the occasional run-in with bears, elk or deer. Running has many different levels, including long distance/marathon, recreational, the short bursts associated with high intensity interval training and track events, and medium to short runs for 5 and 10ks.

But no matter the distance, there are recurring issues that pop up: overuse injuries, sore knees, tight hips and lower back, and weakened forward posture from the constant pounding of one leg's impact on the ground. A balanced, strong body is required to counteract the repetitive effects of running, and that means building a powerful, adaptable and balanced core inside a balanced body. The monotonous striking of feet against ground is absorbed into the ankles, knees and hip, and that transfers into the hamstrings, glutes, hips and lower back. These tight areas must be regularly stretched, strengthened and released for optimum, pain-free running.

Thankfully, Pilates lengthens, stretches and twists your body through flowing dynamic movement. According to RunnersWorld.com, Pilates is essential for the runner's success: "Every Pilates move targets not just the "six-pack" ab muscles (namely, the rectus abdominis and the obliques), but Pilates is also known for targeting the deep core muscles that support your spine and tapping into other commonly neglected muscles in runners such as the glutes and inner thighs."

Running also challenges your respiratory system, so having powerful breath control and a high level of oxygen uptake are important. Proper breathing helps to sustain your consistency and pace during long runs. The deep abdominal breathing of Pilates keeps your center lifted, maximizes the ability of your body to bring in and process the oxygen exchange, and continually adjusts your posture as your feet feverishly pound the pavement. Good alignment, joint mobility and posture further reduce strain and tension in the body, while bad posture and alignment drain your energy reserves, keeping your body fighting against itself. Good alignment and posture also free up energy to be used towards better, faster, longer and more efficient running.

RUNNING PILATES CONDITIONING WORKOUT

1. Forward Fold Mudra
2. Downward Facing Dog with Walks
3. Scissors 100
4. The Roll Up Saw
5. Spine Stretch
6. Shoulder Bridge with Mudra and Shoulders Under the Body
7. Swimming
8. Push Ups
9. Tree Crunch Leg to Side
10. Rowing Series

SKIING/SNOWBOARDING

I tried snowboarding for the first time one day in Montana, when my best friend bought me a lesson for my birthday. It was a very . . . humbling experience. For five hours, I skidded, fell and tipped over—the amount of balance, precision and core strength required was simply not present in me that day.

Living in Colorado, many of my clients are regulars on the slopes. For many months out of the year, they journey to the higher elevations early in the morning to ride the lifts up the slopes and smoothly slide back down on their skis and snowboards. Success on the slopes requires an injury-resistant and flexible body, one with a strong core.

Most of your time is spent in a squatting position, so it's essential you strengthen the glutes, hamstrings and core. Frequently, the skier or snowboarder's back will also be in a hunched position (providing the least amount of wind resistance) which can do tremendous damage to proper posture and alignment over time. Consistent core training is needed to support the spine, lift the upper body and maintain a balance in the abdominals and lower back. The rounded/rolling back position also collapses the chest, resulting in decreased breath support and causing pain in the neck and upper back from increased stress on the shoulder joints. If this is not corrected, the pain and bad posture will only become worse and your time on the slopes might be limited.

Pilates provides a low impact workout which counteracts the many moguls, jumps and sudden changes of direction encountered on the hills. The skier needs balance and stability for controlled weight transfer through turns and stops. Integrating core power to your edging also means you'll transfer energy down into your skis or board, while engaging the core will also reduce stress and fatigue on your knees, back and hips.

SKIING/SNOWBOARDING PILATES CONDITIONING WORKOUT

1. **Toe Touches**
2. **Chair Pose with Twist**
3. **The Roll Up to Boat/Extended Boat**
4. **The Big 5 Series**
5. **Double Leg Kick**
6. **Side Kick**
7. **Leg Pull Front**
8. **Elephant Planks**
9. **Snake**
10. **Lunge Crunches**

⚽ SOCCER/FOOTBALL

Soccer requires pure cardio endurance for success on the field. Whether it's employing quick, powerful forward sprints, leaping for the ball, kicking the ball, diving (for the ball) or changing directions quickly, you need sufficient oxygen uptake efficiency, a strong, balanced core, and back, hip and hamstring flexibility. Pilates addresses all these key points with an integrated and methodical approach.

The Pilates obsession with deep breathing attached to flowing, precise movement will help you control your breath during intense high intensity plays and help with recovery. The more oxygen you pump into your body, the more clarity and endurance you'll have on the field. The stronger and more flexible your core, the more movement potential and agility you'll bring to the game. Building your core—and keeping it strong—also reduces your risk of injury from playing with poor alignment and posture.

Finally, soccer players can suffer from chronic tightness in the hips, hamstrings and lower back. Pilates focuses on strengthening the low back, stretching the hamstrings and lengthening and releasing the hips. Increase range of motion, movement efficiency and cardio performance in your matches/games with a regular Pilates practice.

SOCCER/FOOTBALL
PILATES CONDITIONING WORKOUT

1. Scissors 100
2. Roll Up Mudra
3. The Big 5 Series
4. Swan Dive
5. Scissors
6. Side Kick
7. Teaser
8. Boomerang
9. Elephant Planks
10. Superman Banana

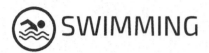 SWIMMING

Pilates and swimming have much in common—fitness disciplines from another mother, you could say. Both are low impact and easy on the joints; they strengthen while stretching through a wide range of movement and motion; they require a full body muscular integration to properly execute the movements; and they both aim to create long, lean, lengthened, and strong bodies while constantly decompressing the spine. Pilates even has several exercises which mimic (and are named after) swimming strokes, which you will find in the playlist below.

In swimming, the core muscles are the basis for all movement. For a swimmer, a strong core will help keep the scapula, pelvis, shoulders and spine/back balanced, structured and aligned. This will make lifting the arms up and out of the water easier without adding strain to the neck muscles. The less strain you can place on your body while cruising through chlorinated water, the better. Pilates teaches your body to move smooth and efficiently so you can store up extra energy and unleash it in the water when needed.

Pilates also trains your body to move in rhythm, synchronized with the breath for greater endurance, efficiency and precision. This translates beautifully to your swimming strokes and your ability to effectively turn your focus to body position, breathing and balance. Train your body to move with the greatest ease and flow. You will swim longer, faster and better with less effort.

SWIMMING
PILATES CONDITIONING WORKOUT

1. Scorpion
2. Pilates 100
3. The Roll Over
4. Swan Dive
5. Shoulder Bridge
6. Jackknife
7. Swimming
8. Leg Pull with Mountain Climbers
9. Backstroke
10. Reverse Swimming

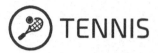# TENNIS

"I started doing Pilates a few weeks ago, which I think has already helped. I did three or four Pilates sessions and my body feels good compared to the last few years when I've come here."

—ANDY MURRAY

Tennis is one of my favorite sports and one I plan to participate in for the rest of my life. It targets both sides of the body with forehands and backhands (though we invariably favor the forehand). Add in the powerful overhead serve, and it's clear why tennis is a forehand-dominated sport.

It's easy to get caught up in predominantly using the forehand because of the extra power we can create when slamming the ball across the court, causing our opponent to change direction, sprint, dive, and miss a just-out-of-reach ball. But rotational force and power must be applied evenly to both sides of the body for healthy balance and alignment, and Pilates is an excellent method for training our bodies to do so efficiently.

Stopping and starting from short bursts of sprints, another core element of tennis, is very challenging; a well-trained and balanced core is needed to pivot the body quickly in many different and unpredictable directions. The body must also be positioned properly before returning the ball over the net, and that takes a high level of agility, speed, precision and coordination. Often, shots are done on the run with one leg off the ground, facing away from the opponent, or even while diving for the ball. Pilates trains the body to react to the unexpected without strain or wasted movement, which will give you an incredible edge on the court.

Effective breathing is needed for powerful and accurate shots and to satisfy the body's need for oxygen during the constant sprinting, jumping, rotating, backwards running and hand-eye coordination that tennis demands.

Tennis is also a very challenging mental game. Matches can last many hours with just you, the racket and your opponent squaring off in a death match, sending the ball sailing over the net to areas which are hopefully unreachable. I played tennis in high school, and the hardest part for me was keeping my mind focused and my emotions in check. I lost several matches because my emotions got the best of me. I talked myself out of playing well and became angrier with every ball I sent into the net or outside the lines. The use of Pilates breath allows you to stay 100% in the match and play at your highest level.

TENNIS PILATES
CONDITIONING WORKOUT

1. Cobra/Updog
2. Boat 100
3. The Roll Up with Twist
4. Rolling like a Ball
5. The Big 5 Series
6. Leg Pull Front
7. Rocking
8. Coordination
9. Backstroke
10. Kick Throughs

VOLLEYBALL/BEACH VOLLEYBALL

I had the honor of attending a college volleyball tournament while presenting at a fitness conference this past spring and was impressed by the raw power, athleticism and body/social awareness they possessed. The way the whole team worked together, constantly moving and flowing to smoothly bump, set and spike the ball was inspiring. Volleyball players need a strong, flexible and stable core which radiates up into the arms and legs to ensure quick control and bursts of power for serving, spiking and bumping.

Volleyball dominates the serving and striking side of a player's body, so it's important to balance the strength through both sides with the full body conditioning of Pilates. When one side prevails in power and strength, your natural alignment and posture deteriorates. You will enjoy better longevity in volleyball by maintaining a balanced and evenly conditioned body.

Because players must be in a constant forward squat position (or digging) to receive the serve, a position which favors the quads and rolls the chest and shoulders forward, constricted posture is a common complaint. To counteract this, a strong postural lift must be applied with Pilates to bring the body back into alignment. This way, players learn to stay lifted when in the forward squat pose.

Word on the street is that beach volleyball legend and Olympic champion, Kerri Walsh Jennings, is obsessed with Pilates and squeezes in Pilates sessions any chance she gets. She practices Pilates regularly to become a more efficient player while building a stronger core and improving her balance. When an athlete at the top of her game like Kerri swears by it, you better take notice!

VOLLEYBALL PILATES CONDITIONING WORKOUT

1. Flop Downs
2. Arms Overhead 100
3. The Roll Up to Extended Boat
4. Single Straight Leg Stretch
5. Double Leg Stretch
6. Swan Dive
7. Double Leg Kick
8. Push Ups
9. Snake
10. Spider Man Burpees

WRESTLING

I wrestled for two years in junior high. Our practices were *brutal*: non-stop wrestling and grappling, followed by running, running and more running. We ran sprints, stairs, long distance . . . I still remember the cotton mouth and gasping for breath. (At the time, I was never properly hydrated nor was my diet on point; my body was always fighting against these deficiencies, but when you're 12–14 years old, the body is more forgiving.) We wrestled and practiced take downs, rolls and ways to dominate and escape your opponents, but the one thing we never did was practice core, flexibility and balance training—three aspects which fill in all the missing pieces and give the wrestler the tools to compete at the highest levels.

Pilates core training is vital to performance when it comes to grappling and wrestling. A stronger and more flexible core makes it much harder to be turned over, controlled or taken down. Huge amounts of core strength are needed to work from a strong position when on the mat and in need of a reversal or escape. A balanced and strong core transfers power, strength and control through the upper and lower body to create a balanced wrestler and shore up any weak spots. This amounts to greater power and endurance throughout the hips, legs, arms and shoulders.

Pilates also helps build flexibility and mobility in the hips, legs, low back, chest and shoulders, preventing injury and keeping the spine decompressed and lengthened when it's placed in the many unexpected positions that occur during a match. From an offensive position, a loose and lithe wrestler will be able to more effectively attack from different positions and add to their repertoire of maneuvers. Defensively, the wrestler is better at countering their opponent's attacks and moves with greater efficiency and control when working from a strong, flexible core. This extra flexibility makes it easier to escape from pins and prolong your wrestling career at a high level of performance.

WRESTLING PILATES CONDITIONING WORKOUT

1. Lunge with Twist
2. Single Leg Stretch 100
3. Rolling like a Ball
4. The Big 5 Series
5. Corkscrew
6. Shoulder Bridge
7. Teaser
8. The Crab
9. Downdog Leg Lifts
10. Superman Burpees

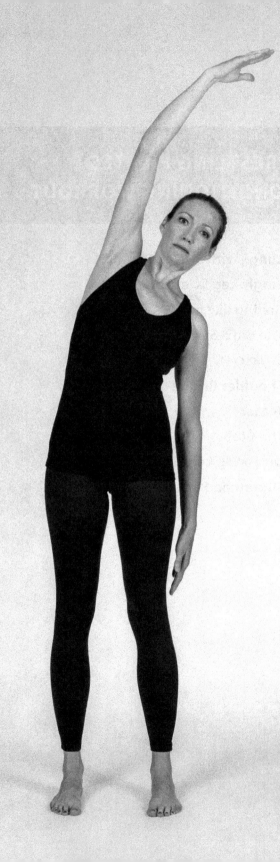

Conclusion

And there you have it! I have trouble artfully expressing the sheer necessity and power of Pilates in words. Words can never be enough—Pilates is *movement*. It is movement, happening right now. Only through the graceful exercises of this thorough conditioning program can we fully understand the direction we must go for optimum athletic performance and improvement.

Train hard. Train smart. Train consistently. Your Pilates practice is a living, breathing organism which gives back what you put in. Once your body gets a taste of the phenomenal improvements to your athletic performance, there is no turning back. Use these exercises, flows and words to enhance your daily training—to enhance your daily life!

Pilates is waiting for you on the mat. So drop down, get into position, take a deep breath, and never look back.

"In 10 sessions, you'll feel the difference; in 20 sessions, you'll see a difference; and in 30 sessions, you'll have a whole new body."
   —Joseph Pilates

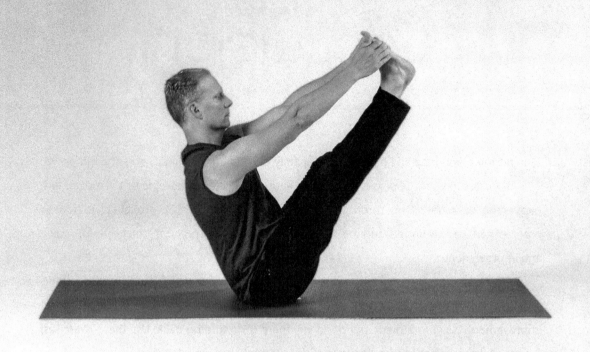

Frequently Asked Questions (FAQs)

Are Pilates and yoga the same thing?

This is easily the most common question I receive regarding Pilates, and the answer is simple: nope! Pilates mat is a system of exercises performed with repetitions and counting, while yoga is a practice comprised of poses (asanas) which are held and sequenced together into flows. They work beautifully *together*, however, as the core focus of Pilates enhances and strengthens yoga poses while the breath and awareness of yoga helps elevate Pilates movements. Even though this book focuses primarily on Pilates, I recommend setting aside time to mix the two disciplines together to further your athletic and mental studies.

If you'd like additional guidance on how to incorporate yoga into your fitness routine, might I suggest my previous book, *Power Yoga for Athletes*?

Will Pilates make me taller?

This is a myth. Pilates will not artificially increase your height, but it *will* help bring you back to your natural height. Factors such as stress, a weak core, bad alignment and uneven posture can decrease our height by pushing our bodies out of alignment, weakening our core support and rolling our shoulders forward. Pilates' focus on core building and body lengthening goes a long way to keeping our bodies tall, strong and balanced.

Does Pilates build muscle?

Pilates focuses on lengthening and strengthening the muscles with constant dynamic movement, leading to the development of long, lean musculature. The goal is to strengthen and elevate both your inner and outer frame while pushing the limits of your mental and physical capacity . . . meaning it won't appreciably increase your muscle mass.

The quickest way to build more mass is to do moderate to heavy strength training (or any kind of strenuous physical activity) which results in delayed onset muscle soreness (DOMS). DOMS is the process of creating tiny tears in your muscles after pushing yourself to your limits in a workout. This discomfort occurs around 24–48 hours after the workout and forces your muscles to rebuild stronger and, often, larger.

Can you get the same workout on the mat as you can with the machines/apparatus?

Pilates on the mat was Joseph Pilates' personal favorite. Through the power of the mind and breath, constant and sufficient tension can be applied throughout all the mat exercises (and the variations, add-ons and modifications in this book!) Training using only a mat also increases the number of exercises that can be performed in a certain amount of time, more effectively adapts to your natural range of motion, and is overall super as you can take your practice anywhere and train at any time.

Didn't Joseph Pilates design Pilates (Contrology) to train only dancers and women?

Joseph Pilates was a boxer, a martial artist and an avid cigar smoker. He designed the Pilates method for optimal physical and mental performance for anyone who would venture into his New York City studio in the 1920s. It so happens that the modern dance explosion was happening in the city at that time, and many dancers flocked to his studio to reap the benefits he was offering. But the power of Pilates is such that no one can keep it a secret and word of mouth spread, proclaiming the life-changing physical benefits this mind/body method offers.

ACKNOWLEDGEMENTS

Thank you eternally to my mom, Beverly, for all her love, support, inspiring phone chats (usually about classic movies, Columbo and books) and gentle voice. I love you, always and forever.

To my BFFs, Peter and Stephan, for all the laughs, ideas, movie quotes and never-ending love and friendship. You guys are the best.

A big thank you to Ryan, Ryan and Andy at Hatherleigh Press, for helping this book become a reality. You guys have been an absolute joy to work with and I'm so pleased with the final product.

Thank you to Kelly Joyce for the fun and creative (16 hour!) photoshoot and your energetic spirit throughout this process.

Thank you to my beautiful wife, Jillian, who was kind enough to model for the book you're holding; our delightful baby Dane, who will be featured in an upcoming book; and our fur baby, Addie. Our mountain family is a constant source of joy, love and inspiration. I love you all.

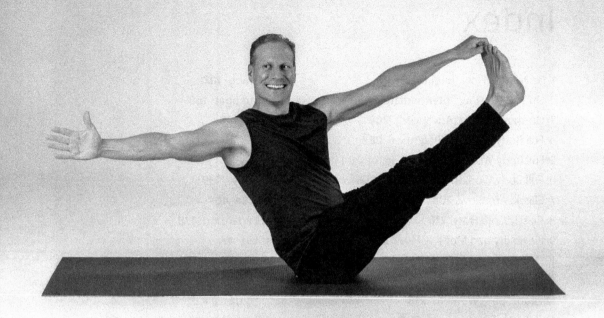

About the Author

SEAN VIGUE is one of the most followed yoga, Pilates, power yoga, flexibility training and performance enhancing instructors in the world, with millions of followers in every corner of the world from beginners to elite professional athletes. He is a bestselling author, including his last major release, *Power Yoga for Athletes*, and greatly enjoys creating books which are accessible to everyone regardless of age and fitness level. Sean has produced thousands of online workout videos, a full DVD line, and his own podcast, and loves teaching at fitness conferences. The more he works in the health and fitness field, the more excited and motivated he gets.

In his spare time he is an amateur film, opera and classical music historian and MST3K fanatic.

Index

Your Pilates Training Journal